WOMEN WITH ADHD

WOMEN'S JOURNEY TO SELF-COMPASSION, CONFIDENCE, AND EMPOWERMENT

RACHEL WRIGHT

WOMEN WITH ADHD

Why You Should Read This Book

Are you a woman seeking empowerment, personal growth, and a deeper understanding of your journey with ADHD?

In a world that often misunderstands ADHD, and particularly how it manifests in women, "Women with ADHD: Women's Journey to Self-Compassion, Confidence, and Empowerment" is the empowering guide you've been searching for. This illuminating book serves as a beacon of understanding and enlightenment on your journey, breaking the chains of stigma, and celebrating the unique strengths that come with being a woman with ADHD.

Discover the reality of ADHD, one that transcends the misconceptions and stereotypes. Recognize ADHD not as a disability, but as a different way of processing the world – a unique lens that can offer incredible insights, creativity, and problem-solving abilities. The book starts by unveiling the often-hidden strengths of ADHD, transforming the perceived 'chaos' into a source of power and inspiration.

In this essential guide, **you'll navigate through personal stories of women who've walked the same path, women who've harnessed the power of ADHD to excel in various facets of life.** You'll be welcomed into the 'Sisterhood of ADHD', a community of understanding, support, and collective growth. This connection will remind you that you're not alone, and will encourage you to draw strength from shared experiences.

You'll also delve into practical strategies for managing ADHD. **This book provides actionable steps for you to not only survive but truly thrive.** You'll learn effective treatments, coping mechanisms, and life skills that cater specifically to women with ADHD. Explore various strategies on how to flourish in relationships, thrive in the workplace, and create a self-care sanctuary that respects and accommodates your unique needs.

Perhaps the most transformative part of your journey will be self-understanding and self-empowerment. This book illuminates the path to a deeper understanding of your unique traits, helping you embrace and nurture your individuality. **It encourages you to unleash your 'superpowers', turning the perceived challenges of ADHD into sources of strength and resilience.**

This book equips you to become an advocate for yourself and others with ADHD. It offers a guide to lighting the way, empowering you to become a beacon of hope, understanding, and acceptance in your communities.

Every page of this book is a testament to the strength, resilience, and immense potential of women with ADHD. It serves as a reminder that your neurodiversity is not a burden to be managed but a unique strength to be harnessed and celebrated. If you are a woman living with ADHD or know someone who does, this book is an invaluable resource, a companion that will inspire you to embrace your unique journey and unlock the extraordinary potential that lies within.

In "Women with ADHD: Women's Journey to Self-Compassion, Confidence, and Empowerment," you're not just reading a book – you're embarking on an empowering journey of self-discovery and growth.

It's time to stop merely surviving and start thriving. Unleash your potential and redefine what it means to be a woman with ADHD.

Thank You!

Thank you for your purchase.

I am dedicated to making the most enriching and informational content. I hope it meets your expectations and you gain a lot from it.

Your comments and feedback are important to me because they help me to provide the best material possible.

Again, thank you for your purchase.

INTRODUCTION

"In diversity there is beauty and there is strength." - Maya Angelou

Welcome to a transformative journey of empowerment and self-discovery. Within the pages of this book, we'll embark on a remarkable exploration of the unique experiences, challenges, and strengths of women with ADHD (attention-deficit/hyperactivity disorder). This book is a beacon of hope, a guide to embracing your true potential, and a celebration of the amazing resilience and brilliance that lies within you.

Before we dive into the heart of this empowering journey, let me express my gratitude for your presence here. By choosing to engage with this book, you've taken a powerful step toward understanding, growth, and self-empowerment. Your decision to explore the world of ADHD and its impact on women isn't only an act of self-care but also an investment in your personal development and well-being.

This book is a follow-up to my previous work, titled *Women with ADHD Falling through the Cracks: Unmasking the Bias and Exploring Why ADD and ADHD Symptoms in Adult Women and Girls Are Misunderstood and Undiagnosed*. In that book, we delved into the complex factors contributing to the underdiagnosis and misunderstanding of ADHD in women and girls. We uncovered the biases, stereotypes, and societal barriers that hindered their journey toward recognition and support.

Building upon that foundation, this book takes us further on the path of empowerment and self-care. It aims to provide you, as a woman with ADHD, with the knowledge, strategies, and inspiration to embrace your uniqueness, navigate the challenges that come with ADHD, and create a life of fulfillment, purpose, and success.

In the chapters that follow, we'll engage in a multidimensional exploration of your journey with ADHD. We'll delve into the hidden strengths that often accompany ADHD, debunk misconceptions and stigmas, and showcase real-life stories of women who've harnessed their ADHD to achieve personal and professional success. We'll investigate the female experience of ADHD, exploring the unique challenges faced by women and uncovering strategies for overcoming hurdles. We'll come to appreciate the power of community, the importance of self-understanding, and the transformative impact of self-care. Moreover, we'll dive into the realm of advocacy that will empower you to become a champion for yourself and others, foster understanding, and ignite positive change.

Imagine a world where women with ADHD fully embrace their power, recognize their unique strengths, and thrive in all aspects of their lives. This book is here to remind you that such a world is within your reach. It's a testament to the powerful potential that lies within you and a guide to unlocking that potential.

At times, the journey of a woman with ADHD can feel

like navigating uncharted waters. Societal expectations, internal struggles, and lack of understanding can create a sense of isolation and frustration. However, within those challenges lie hidden treasures waiting to be discovered. It's time to embark on a transformative journey of self-discovery, self-acceptance, and empowerment.

As we delve into the chapters ahead, you'll come to realize that having ADHD isn't a flaw or a limitation but a unique aspect of your identity. It brings with it a set of strengths that, when harnessed, can propel you to great heights. Creativity, intuition, hyperfocus, and a unique perspective on the world are just a few examples of the extraordinary abilities that often accompany ADHD. It's time to embrace these strengths and embrace the radiant power within you.

This book isn't just a collection of theories and research findings. It's a tapestry woven of personal stories, strategies, and practical guidance from women who've walked a similar path. Their journeys will inspire and guide you as you navigate the twists and turns of your own ADHD journey. You're not alone in this. You're part of a vibrant community of women who are rising above societal expectations, defying stereotypes, and forging their own path to success and fulfillment.

Knowledge is the key that unlocks the door to empowerment. As we embark on this journey together, we must arm ourselves with a deep understanding of ADHD and its unique impact on women. By gaining knowledge, we can dispel myths, challenge misconceptions, and pave the way for greater understanding and support.

In the following chapters, we'll explore the intricacies of ADHD, its varieties, symptoms, and how it manifests differently in females than in males. We'll delve into the factors contributing to the underdiagnosis and misunderstanding of ADHD in women and girls. By shining a light on these issues, we can create a foundation of knowledge that will empower you to navigate your journey with clarity and confidence.

Understanding the complexities of ADHD isn't just about self-awareness. It's also about fostering empathy and compassion within ourselves and in the broader society. By sharing this knowledge with others, we can break down barriers, challenge stigmas, and encourage a more inclusive and sympathetic environment for women with ADHD.

As you absorb the information within these pages, remember that knowledge isn't static. It's a journey of continuous learning and growth. The field of ADHD research and understanding is constantly evolving, and new insights are being discovered. Stay curious, stay informed, and continue to educate yourself to deepen your knowledge of ADHD.

The journey of empowerment begins with a call to action. It's an invitation to embrace your unique journey with ADHD and step into your power as a woman who's capable of achieving greatness. This book serves as a guidebook, providing the tools, strategies, and inspiration to unleash your true potential.

Empowerment isn't a passive process. It requires active engagement, self-reflection, and a commitment to personal growth. It's about acknowledging your strengths, embracing your challenges, and taking intentional steps toward creating a life filled with purpose, fulfillment, and self-care.

Throughout this book, we'll explore various aspects of empowerment—from building resilience to nurturing self-compassion, cultivating healthy relationships, and advocating for yourself and others. Each chapter is designed to provide you with insights, practical strategies, and real-life examples to guide you on this transformative journey.

It's important to remember that empowerment is a personal and unique journey. Your path may differ from that of others, and that's perfectly okay. Embrace your individuality, honor your journey, and allow yourself to evolve and grow at your own pace. Your empowerment isn't a destination but a continuous process of self-discovery and self-actualization.

As we embark on this journey together, I invite you to approach each chapter with an open mind and an open heart. Be curious, be willing to challenge yourself, and be receptive to the transformative power that lies within you. Let's walk the path of empowerment by celebrating our strengths, supporting one another, and lighting the way for women with ADHD worldwide.

Throughout the chapters ahead, we will explore the multifaceted aspects of women's experiences with ADHD. We'll celebrate the triumphs, navigate the setbacks, and embrace the power of self-care and advocacy.

Remember that this book isn't a quick fix or a magic solution. It's a guidebook to accompany you as you navigate the complexities of your journey with ADHD. It will provide you with knowledge, strategies, and stories of inspiration to empower you along the way. However, ultimately, the power to transform your life lies within you.

So, we're now ready to begin this transformative journey together. Let's embrace our ADHD, honor our strengths, and rise above societal expectations. Let's support one another, celebrate our unique journeys, and create a world where women with ADHD are seen, understood, and empowered.

The gratifying journey awaits. Are you ready to embrace it?

CHAPTER 1: UNEARTHING THE HIDDEN STRENGTHS OF ADHD

As we embark on this journey, the first step is to delve deeper into understanding the true nature of ADHD. Attention-deficit/hyperactivity disorder, or ADHD, is a neurodevelopmental disorder that affects both children and adults. It's often characterized by persistent patterns of inattention, hyperactivity, and impulsivity. It's a condition that's often misunderstood and has numerous misconceptions.

ADHD isn't just about being easily distracted or hyperactive. It's also not exclusive to childhood or a disorder that people "grow out of." It's not a label for unruly behavior or the result of poor parenting or lack of discipline. And most importantly, it's not a defining limitation.

In reality, ADHD is a different way of thinking. It's characterized by a unique wiring of the brain that creates its own set of challenges but also has unique strengths. Yes, you read that right—strengths. In this chapter, we'll investigate these hidden strengths that often go unnoticed or underappreciated.

ADHD, for all its challenges, can bestow individuals with unique attributes. Many women with ADHD are remarkably creative. Their minds, buzzing with activity, can be fertile ground for innovation and originality. Their divergent thinking can lead them to find novel solutions to problems, and their non-linear thought processes can often result in unique perspectives. This creativity can manifest in various fields—from art and literature to science and technology—and has contributed to significant advancements and achievements.

Another common trait among women with ADHD is their heightened empathy. They tend to be deeply attuned to the emotions of others and capable of profound compassion and understanding. This allows them to be excellent friends, partners, and caregivers because they can forge deep, meaningful relationships. They're often attracted to professions and causes where they can use their empathy to make a difference, such as counseling, social work, activism, and more.

Resilience is yet another strength often found in women with ADHD. Living with ADHD in a world that doesn't fully understand or accommodate it can be challenging. However, it's precisely these challenges that forge the resilience and determination that many women with ADHD possess. They're fighters and survivors who learn to adapt and persevere in the face of adversity. They learn to turn their challenges into stepping stones, using them to grow stronger and build a life of success and fulfillment.

Let's take a moment to look at some real-life examples of this resilience and success. Consider the story of Simone Biles, the world-renowned gymnast who's won numerous Olympic gold medals. Biles has been open about her ADHD diagnosis and has used her platform to challenge the stigma surrounding the condition. Despite the challenges that ADHD poses, she's harnessed her ability to hyperfocus—a common ADHD trait—to excel in her sport. Her story is a testament to the fact that ADHD doesn't limit one's potential for greatness.

Or, consider the story of Lisa Ling, a celebrated journalist and TV presenter who was diagnosed with ADHD as an adult. She's spoken about how her ADHD has been a challenge for her but also about how it's contributed to her success as a journalist. Her relentless curiosity, her ability to go deep into her news stories, and her unique perspective are all traits that she attributes to her ADHD.

These are just two examples of the many women who've harnessed their ADHD to achieve great things. They've used unique ADHD attributes—creativity, empathy, and resilience—as tools for achieving success. They've learned to see their ADHD not as a limitation but as a strength.

As we move forward on this journey, remember these stories and these strengths. Remember that ADHD is more than the challenges it presents; it's a unique way of experiencing the world that comes with its own set of gifts. In the coming chapters, we'll delve deeper into these strengths, exploring ways to harness and use them to your advantage.

One of the most significant advantages of ADHD is its ability to allow an individual to hyperfocus. Hyperfocus refers to intense concentration and absorption in a particular task or activity. Although the attention of a person with ADHD may drift in situations that are mundane or lack stimulation, when something captures the interest of an individual with ADHD, they can zone in on it with an almost unparalleled intensity. This ability to hyperfocus can lead to periods of intense productivity and deep dives into areas of interest. Hyperfocusing can be a powerful tool when directed toward constructive activities, and many successful women with ADHD have used it to excel in their field.

Women with ADHD also possess remarkable adaptability. Given the right environment and support, they can easily adjust to changes and transitions. This ability to adapt stems from their experience navigating a world not always designed for their unique brain wiring. It's a skill that can be tremendously beneficial in our rapidly evolving world in which change is the only constant.

In addition, many women with ADHD exhibit exceptional intuition. Their brains are constantly absorbing information, processing cues, and making connections. This often leads to a heightened sense of knowing, allowing them to "read" situations or people accurately. This can be an invaluable asset in personal relationships and professional scenarios alike.

Finally, many women with ADHD display boundless energy and enthusiasm that can be infectious. When channeled productively, this energy can be a driving force that propels them toward their goals and positively influences those around them.

However, it's important to note that these strengths don't negate the challenges of ADHD. They're two sides of the same coin; acknowledging one doesn't mean disregarding the other. This book aims to provide a holistic understanding of ADHD—recognizing its struggles and celebrating the strengths.

The stories and strengths discussed in this chapter lay

the foundation for the rest of this book. As we delve deeper into the practicalities of living with ADHD, remember these strengths. Remember the creativity, the empathy, the resilience, the hyperfocus, the adaptability, the intuition, and the energy that are often associated with ADHD. Remember the stories of women who've harnessed these strengths to carve out successful and fulfilling lives.

Now let's move forward, armed with the knowledge of the hidden strengths of ADHD and the determination to harness them to their fullest potential.

CHAPTER 2: JOURNEY INTO THE UNSEEN: WOMEN CONFRONTING ADHD

ADHD is an equal-opportunity condition in that it affects people of all ages, genders, and walks of life. However, for many years, research focus on ADHD has been skewed toward a single demographic—young boys. This has led to a widespread belief that ADHD is a disorder of prepubescent males, resulting in many girls and women with ADHD going undiagnosed and unsupported.

This chapter aims to shine a light on the unseen journey of women with ADHD, exploring the unique ways the condition presents in women and the distinct challenges they face. The goal of this exploration isn't just to inform and educate but to provide a sense of validation and community for women living with ADHD. You're not alone in your journey; your experiences are seen and validated.

ADHD in females often looks different than it does in males. While hyperactivity and impulsivity are hallmark symptoms of ADHD, they're more commonly observed in boys and men than in girls and women. Women with ADHD often exhibit symptoms of inattention that can include difficulty focusing, forgetfulness, disorganization, and struggles with time management.

These symptoms are often mistaken for personality traits or quirks rather than signs of a neurodevelopmental disorder. A woman who's constantly losing her keys, forgetting appointments, or struggling to stay organized may be labeled as forgetful or careless. Her struggles are often internalized as personal failures, leading to a cycle of self-blame and lowered self-esteem.

Moreover, women are often socialized to be people-pleasers and caregivers, leading many women with ADHD to develop coping mechanisms to hide their symptoms. They may work twice as hard to stay organized, often at the expense of their mental and physical health. They may overcompensate in areas they find challenging, leading to burnout and exhaustion.

The societal pressure to conform to gender norms can exacerbate the struggles of women with ADHD. Women are often expected to be the organizers and caretakers, roles that can be especially challenging for those with ADHD. The inability to meet these expectations can lead to feelings of inadequacy and shame.

Additionally, hormonal changes throughout a woman's life can significantly impact the severity of ADHD symptoms. Fluctuations in estrogen levels during menstrual cycles, pregnancy, and menopause can exacerbate ADHD behaviors, adding an additional layer of complexity to a woman's experience with ADHD.

All these factors contribute to a unique presentation of

ADHD in women, and its symptoms are often overlooked or misunderstood. However, with growing awareness, the tide is slowly changing. More and more women are being diagnosed with ADHD and receiving the support they need.

The journey of a woman with ADHD may be fraught with challenges, but it's also a journey that leads to resilience and empowerment. It's a journey of learning to navigate a neurotypical world with a neurodivergent brain. It's a journey of learning to celebrate your unique brain wiring rather than seeing it as a deficit.

As we proceed on this journey in the following chapters, remember that your experiences are valid. Your struggles aren't personal failures but the result of a brain that's wired differently. This different wiring can become a unique strength with a correct understanding and support.

Obtaining a diagnosis of ADHD as a woman can be a challenging process. Given the misconceptions and stereotypes surrounding ADHD, many women go undiagnosed until adulthood. Some may go their entire lives without knowing they have ADHD, attributing their struggles to personal shortcomings rather than a neurodevelopmental condition.

The diagnostic process often begins with recognizing the symptoms. This could be spurred by a variety of things. Perhaps you read an article about ADHD in women, or a friend or family member suggests the possibility. Maybe you see your own struggles mirrored in your child after they've been diagnosed with ADHD.

Once the seed of suspicion has been planted, the next step is seeking professional help. Given the stigma surrounding mental health, this can often be a daunting process. But remember, seeking help isn't a sign of weakness. It's an act of courage and self-care. It's the first step toward better understanding yourself and controlling your ADHD.

When seeking a diagnosis, you may encounter healthcare professionals who aren't well-versed in recognizing the symptoms of ADHD in women. You may face dismissal or invalidation of your struggles. This is where self-advocacy comes into play. It's crucial to remember that you know yourself best. If you believe you may have ADHD, don't be afraid to seek a second opinion or ask for a referral to a specialist.

Receiving a diagnosis of ADHD can often elicit a mix of emotions. There may be relief at finally having an explanation for your struggles but also fear and uncertainty about what comes next. This is a normal part of the process, and it's essential to give yourself permission to feel these emotions.

One essential aspect of navigating life with ADHD is self-care. Women, especially, often find themselves in caregiving roles, prioritizing the needs of others over their own. However, it's important to remember that you can't pour from an empty cup.

Self-care for women with ADHD might look slightly different than self-care for other women. It's not just about bubble baths and spa days but about creating routines and structures that cater to your ADHD brain. It's about setting boundaries and learning to say no. It's about seeking support when you need it and being compassionate with yourself when things don't go as planned.

To provide a more tangible understanding of receiving and living with a diagnosis of ADHD, let's hear from some women who've walked this path. Consider the story of Sarah, a successful entrepreneur who was diagnosed with ADHD in her late thirties. For Sarah, receiving this diagnosis was like finding the missing piece of a puzzle. It helped her understand why she struggled with things that seemed to come easily to others. With her diagnosis, she was able to seek the proper support and strategies to manage her ADHD, leading to a significant improvement in her quality of life.

Or consider the story of Priya, a professor who was diagnosed with ADHD in her early twenties. Priya always knew she was different, but she couldn't pinpoint why. She was smart and creative but struggled with organization and time management. Her ADHD diagnosis came as a relief, providing an explanation for her struggles. It also led her to discover a community of women with similar experiences that helped her feel seen and understood.

These stories are a testament to the resilience and strength of women with ADHD. They showcase the power of understanding and embracing your ADHD and turning what's often seen as a deficit into a unique strength.

In this chapter, we explored the unseen journey of women with ADHD, delving into their unique challenges and the resilience they showcase. As we move forward, we'll explore strategies and resources to manage ADHD, highlighting the importance of self-advocacy and self-care.

In understanding the unique challenges women with ADHD face, it's also important to address the stigma and misconceptions surrounding the condition. Unfortunately, despite advancements in science and awareness, ADHD is often trivialized or dismissed as lacking discipline or willpower. This lack of understanding can lead to feelings of isolation and self-doubt in women with ADHD.

Therefore, one of the goals of this book—and this chapter, in particular—is to debunk these misconceptions. ADHD is a medically acknowledged neurodevelopmental condition that affects all aspects of life. Coping with ADHD isn't a matter of trying harder or being more disciplined. Finding the strengths in living with ADHD begins with accepting that you have a brain that's wired differently and learning to take advantage of this different wiring to your benefit.

It's also essential to emphasize that having ADHD doesn't limit your potential or define your worth. Many successful women have ADHD, from entrepreneurs and artists to scientists and authors. They've harnessed their ADHD to fuel their creativity, drive, and resilience, carving out successful and fulfilling lives.

Having ADHD simply means that you experience the world differently. It means you're *different,* not *defective.* With this understanding, you can shift your perspective of ADHD to see it as a part of who you are rather than a problem to be fixed.

Throughout this journey, remember that you're not alone. Millions of women around the world are walking the same path. There are communities and resources available to support you, some of which we'll explore in the coming chapters.

In the next chapter, we'll discuss practical strategies and tools to manage ADHD. We'll explore topics such as organization, time management, self-care, and more. These strategies aren't about changing who you are but about creating an environment that supports you.

Before we move on, take a moment to reflect on the information shared in this chapter. How does it resonate with your experience? What emotions does it evoke? Remember, there's no right or wrong way to feel. Your journey is unique to you, and all your feelings are valid.

As we continue this journey of understanding and embracing ADHD, carry these stories and insights with you. Let them be a source of strength and validation. Remember, you're seen, you're valued, and you're not alone.

CHAPTER 3: TAMING THE CHAOS: PRACTICAL STRATEGIES FOR MANAGING ADHD

ADHD isn't a one-size-fits-all condition. It manifests differently in different people, shaped by gender, age, personality, and life experiences. Therefore, the management of ADHD is also not a one-size-fits-all strategy. A management plan must be tailored to fit each individual's unique strengths and challenges. This chapter aims to provide a toolkit of strategies that can be adapted and personalized to fit your unique ADHD journey.

One of the key challenges for many women with ADHD is organization. The ADHD brain thrives in chaos, often leading to cluttered spaces and disorganized schedules. External chaos can often lead to internal chaos, exacerbating ADHD symptoms. Therefore, developing organizational strategies that are aligned with your ADHD brain is crucial.

Start by creating an ADHD-friendly environment. This could mean having a designated place for everything, using visual cues such as labels and color-coding, or creating a clutter-free workspace. Remember, the goal isn't to create a perfectly organized space that could be featured in a "better living" magazine but a functional space that supports your ADHD brain.

Next, consider using tools and apps to enhance organization and time management. These might include digital calendars, reminder apps, or project-management tools. Experiment with different tools to find what works best for you. Remember, the most effective tool is the one you actually use, so choose something that aligns with your preferences and lifestyle.

Creating routines can also be helpful in managing ADHD. Routines provide structure and predictability, helping to reduce decision-making fatigue and overwhelm. However, the ADHD brain often resists routine, regarding it as boring or restrictive. Therefore, it's important to create flexible routines that incorporate variety and novelty.

For example, you could create a morning routine that includes several activities such as exercise, meditation, and journaling. You can mix and match these activities based on your mood and energy level to provide the novelty your ADHD brain craves while still maintaining a semblance of routine.

Don't underestimate the power of small, incremental changes. You don't have to overhaul your entire life at once. Start small, choose one area to focus on, and gradually build on your successes. Celebrate your progress, no matter how small, and remember that progress isn't always linear. There will be setbacks, but that's part of the journey.

Managing ADHD isn't just about focusing and organization. This complex condition can affect all aspects of your life, including your emotions, relationships, and self-esteem. Therefore, managing

ADHD isn't just about implementing organizational strategies; it's also about taking care of your emotional and mental health.

Self-care is crucial to managing ADHD, but it often gets overlooked, especially by women. Women are often caregivers, prioritizing the needs of others over their own. However, self-care isn't selfish; it's necessary. Remember, you can't pour from an empty cup.

Consider the story of Maria, a mother of two diagnosed with ADHD in her forties. Maria often found herself overwhelmed by the demands of work and family life. She was always putting the needs of others before her own, and she often felt exhausted. After her diagnosis, Maria realized the importance of self-care. She started setting boundaries, prioritizing her needs, and creating routines that supported her ADHD brain. This not only helped her manage her ADHD symptoms but also improved her overall well-being and happiness.

Next, let's talk about emotions. Women with ADHD often experience intense emotions, a symptom known as emotional dysregulation. This can lead to mood swings, impulsive reactions, and feelings of overwhelm. Understanding and managing your emotions is a crucial part of managing ADHD.

Start by recognizing and validating your emotions. Remember, it's okay to feel what you're feeling. Your emotions are valid, and they aren't a sign of weakness.

Next, develop coping strategies that work for you. This could include mindfulness practices, physical activity, creative outlets, or seeking support from a therapist or coach. Remember, it's not only okay but essential to seek help. You don't have to navigate this journey alone.

Finally, let's touch on the topic of relationships. ADHD can impact your relationships in various ways, from struggles with communication to challenges with executive-functioning tasks like household chores. Understanding how ADHD affects your relationships and developing strategies to navigate these challenges is crucial.

Start by having open and honest conversations about your ADHD with your loved ones. Help them understand your struggles and how they can support you. Consider seeking support from a therapist or coach, individually or as a couple or family.

The journey of managing ADHD isn't linear; it involves trial and error, setbacks, and victories. It's a continuous process of self-discovery and learning. As you explore strategies for managing ADHD, keep in mind that what works for one person may not work for you. The key is to keep experimenting, keep learning, and keep adapting.

In professional life, women with ADHD may face unique challenges. You might struggle with staying organized, meeting deadlines, or maintaining focus during long meetings. On the other hand, you might excel at creative problem-solving, thinking outside the box, and bringing enthusiasm and energy to your work.

To navigate the professional world with ADHD, start by understanding your unique strengths and challenges. What aspects of your work do you excel at? Where do you struggle? Once you understand this, you can start to carve out a work environment that supports your ADHD brain.

This could involve using tools and strategies to manage your time and tasks, creating an ADHD-friendly workspace, or seeking special accommodations at work. Remember, it's okay to ask for what you need. You deserve to work in an environment that supports your success.

A significant part of managing ADHD involves leaning into your strengths—such as creativity, empathy, resilience, and the ability to think outside the box. By recognizing and harnessing these strengths, you can transform your ADHD from a challenge into a superpower.

For instance, your creativity and out-of-the-box thinking could make you a brilliant problem-solver. Your empathy could make you a great leader or counselor. Your resilience—born out of navigating a world that's not designed for your ADHD brain—could be your biggest strength.

Once again, managing ADHD is not about fixing yourself or trying to fit into a neurotypical mold. It's about understanding your unique brain wiring and creating a life that supports it. It's about celebrating your strengths, managing challenges, and embracing your unique journey.

Before we move on, take a moment to reflect on the strategies shared in this chapter. Which ones resonated with you? Which ones would you like to try? Remember, there's no right or wrong answer, and you can decide what works best for you.

Next, we'll delve into the power of community and support in managing ADHD.

CHAPTER 4: THE SISTERHOOD OF ADHD

THE SHARED JOURNEY

In this chapter, we'll explore the profound connections and shared experiences that unite women with ADHD. We'll investigate the sisterhood of women with ADHD, recognizing the power of community and the strength that comes from knowing we're not alone.

Living with ADHD can sometimes feel isolating. The challenges we face, the moments of self-doubt, and the internal struggles can disconnect us from those around us. However, within this shared experience lies a remarkable sense of camaraderie and understanding.

49

By coming together as a sisterhood, we can find solace, support, and empowerment.

The journey of ADHD isn't the same for every woman, but there are common threads that weave us together. The experiences of distractibility, impulsivity, and hyperactivity may manifest differently for each of us, but the underlying source of these symptoms is the same. By embracing our shared journey, we tap into a collective strength that helps us navigate the challenges and celebrate the victories.

One of the most powerful aspects of the sisterhood of ADHD is the validation it provides. When we connect with other women who understand our struggles and experiences, we no longer feel we're outliers or misfits. We realize that our challenges aren't personal failings but rather shared aspects of ADHD. This validation allows us to shed the weight of self-judgment and embrace self-compassion. We learn to be kinder to ourselves and to extend that kindness to others within the sisterhood.

The ADHD sisterhood provides a safe space to share our stories, triumphs, and vulnerabilities. It's a community where we can express ourselves authentically without fear of judgment. This shared vulnerability fosters deep connections and allows us to learn from one another's experiences. We gain insights, strategies, and support from women who've walked in our shoes. The power of shared wisdom and collective experiences propels us forward and helps us thrive in a world that may not always understand or accommodate our needs.

The sisterhood of women with ADHD extends beyond geographical boundaries and physical spaces. Thanks to the digital age, we can connect with women from all walks of life, across continents, and create a virtual sisterhood. Online support groups, forums, and social media platforms have become invaluable resources for women with ADHD. They provide a platform to ask questions, seek advice, and share our victories and challenges. The sense of belonging and understanding that comes from these connections is immeasurable, reinforcing the strength and power of the sisterhood.

BUILDING A SUPPORTIVE NETWORK

We touched on the power of the sisterhood of ADHD and the shared journey that unites us. Now, let's delve deeper into the importance of building a supportive network and the role it plays in our lives.

Building a supportive network is essential for our well-being and growth. It provides us with a sense of belonging, understanding, and validation. Surrounding ourselves with individuals who share similar experiences helps to alleviate the sense of isolation and provides a platform for genuine connection. Whether it's in-person support groups, online communities, or close friendships, having a supportive network allows us to lean on one another during challenging times and celebrate each other's successes.

Support groups specifically tailored for women with ADHD can be particularly impactful. These groups provide a space for open and honest conversations about our experiences, challenges, and triumphs. Within these groups, we find solace in knowing that others face similar hurdles and can offer insights and empathy. We're given the opportunity to learn from one another, exchange coping strategies, and find comfort among other individuals who know what our life is like. Whether it's discovering a new time-management technique, a mindfulness practice, or a self-care ritual, the collective wisdom of the sisterhood becomes a treasure trove of knowledge and growth.

In addition to support groups, professional guidance can play a crucial role. Seeking therapy or coaching from professionals specializing in ADHD can provide valuable insights, tools, and personalized strategies for managing our unique challenges. These professionals can help us navigate the intricacies of our ADHD journey, develop coping mechanisms, and empower us to embrace our strengths.

While support groups and professional guidance are vital, the sisterhood of ADHD extends beyond formal settings. Informal connections such as friendships and mentorships are equally important. Finding like-minded individuals who understand and accept us—whether they have ADHD or not—helps to create a network of support in various aspects of our lives.

These connections offer understanding, encouragement, and a sense of camaraderie that contributes to our overall well-being.

SHARING AND LEARNING

The sisterhood of ADHD provides a unique platform for sharing our stories and experiences. By openly sharing our journey, we not only find validation and support but also create opportunities for growth and learning. We inspire and uplift others when we share our triumphs, challenges, and strategies. Likewise, when we listen to the stories of our sisters, we gain new perspectives, insights, and coping mechanisms that can enhance our lives.

Sharing our experiences within the sisterhood allows us to break down the walls of isolation and shame. It liberates us from the burden of hiding our ADHD and invites others to do the same. Being vulnerable and open creates a safe space for others to express themselves authentically. In this space, we can celebrate our strengths, navigate challenges together, and foster a sense of unity and understanding.

Learning from one another is a cornerstone of the sisterhood of ADHD. We all have unique strengths, experiences, and perspectives that can enrich the lives of others. By actively listening and engaging in conversations, we gain valuable insights and strategies to manage our ADHD more effectively.

The act of sharing and learning within the sisterhood goes beyond individual growth. It also contributes to the collective empowerment of women with ADHD. By sharing our stories, we challenge societal misconceptions, raise awareness, and advocate for a more inclusive and understanding world. Together, our voices become a powerful force that fosters change, dismantles stigmas, and empowers other women with ADHD to embrace their true potential.

THE POWER OF EMPATHY

Empathy is the cornerstone of human connection, and within the sisterhood of ADHD, it takes on a special significance. When we encounter others who understand the intricacies of living with ADHD, we experience a profound sense of empathy that may be unlike anything we've ever felt before. This empathy stems from the deep understanding of walking a similar path. It allows us to see beyond the surface and genuinely connect with one another.

The power of empathy lies in its ability to comfort, validate, and empower. When we share our challenges and vulnerabilities within the sisterhood, we find solace in knowing that others have experienced similar struggles. We're no longer alone in our journey, and this understanding brings immense comfort. Moreover, the validation and support we receive through empathy give us the strength to embrace our ADHD, celebrate our strengths, and persevere through the obstacles that may arise.

Empathy within the sisterhood also fosters personal growth and self-acceptance. We learn to extend that same empathy to ourselves when we're regarded with empathy. This self-compassion and understanding lay the foundation for self-acceptance and allow us to embrace our strengths, quirks, and imperfections without judgment.

Additionally, the power of empathy extends beyond

our individual experiences. It drives us to advocate for greater understanding and support for all women with ADHD. By sharing our stories and fostering empathy within the broader society, we challenge the misconceptions, biases, and stereotypes surrounding ADHD. Through empathy, we pave the way for a more inclusive world where women with ADHD are seen, heard, and empowered.

EMBRACING THE STRENGTH OF THE SISTERHOOD

Embracing the strength of the sisterhood means recognizing the power that lies within our shared experiences. When we come together, we create a vibrant tapestry of diverse stories, perspectives, and strengths. This collective strength allows us to tackle challenges, inspire change, and advocate for greater understanding and support.

The sisterhood of ADHD serves as a source of inspiration and encouragement. By witnessing the successes and triumphs of fellow sisters, we believe in our own ability to overcome obstacles and achieve our goals. Whether it's a woman who excels in her career, balances motherhood with ADHD, or creates meaningful change through advocacy, their stories remind us of our own limitless potential.

Within the sisterhood, we find allies and supporters who uplift and champion our endeavors. When we share our dreams, aspirations, and challenges, we're supported by a network of individuals who believe in us and our abilities. This support fuels our motivation, instills resilience, and propels us forward on our personal and professional journeys.

Embracing the strength of the sisterhood also means taking an active role in supporting others. By lifting up our sisters, we create a ripple effect of empowerment and growth. We celebrate their achievements, provide a listening ear during difficult times, and offer guidance and insights when needed. This collective support reinforces the bonds within the sisterhood and creates an environment of collaboration, growth, and mutual respect.

As we embrace the strength of the sisterhood, we're

reminded of the remarkable resilience and brilliance that exists within each and every one of us. We aren't defined by our challenges but by our ability to rise above them. Together, let's continue to nurture the sisterhood of ADHD and create a world where women with ADHD can truly flourish.

CHAPTER 5: THE GIFT OF SELF-UNDERSTANDING

THE SIGNIFICANCE OF SELF-UNDERSTANDING

Understanding oneself is a pivotal step in embracing and managing ADHD. In this chapter, we'll embark on a journey of self-discovery and explore the significance of self-understanding for women with ADHD. By recognizing the signs, overcoming challenges, and embracing our unique identities, we can unlock the gift of self-understanding and find empowerment in our ADHD journey.

Self-understanding is more than just knowing and accepting that we've been diagnosed with ADHD. It involves gaining insight into our strengths, weaknesses, triggers, and unique neurodivergent experiences. By developing self-awareness, we can better comprehend how ADHD affects various aspects of our lives, including relationships, work, and personal well-being. Self-understanding empowers us to make informed decisions, seek appropriate support, and design strategies that align with our individual needs.

Embracing our ADHD as part of our unique identity is a transformative step in our journey of self-understanding. It involves accepting and reframing ADHD as a neurodivergent trait that brings both challenges and strengths. By shifting our perspective and embracing our ADHD identity, we can unleash our potential, tap into our creative abilities, and navigate the world with authenticity and self-compassion.

THE ROAD TO DIAGNOSIS

Recognizing the need for an ADHD evaluation is an

essential step toward self-understanding and accessing appropriate support. If you suspect you may have ADHD based on the symptoms and challenges you experience, it's crucial to trust your instincts and seek professional evaluation from a qualified healthcare provider or mental health professional.

The diagnostic process for ADHD typically involves a complete medical history and a comprehensive assessment that evaluates symptoms and their impact on various areas of the individual's life. This process may include interviews, questionnaires, cognitive assessments, and collaboration with loved ones or significant others who can provide additional insights. It's essential to be open and honest during this process to ensure an accurate diagnosis.

Diagnosing ADHD in women can be more complex due to various factors we've already discussed—societal biases, gender stereotypes, and differences in how symptoms may present. Women often develop coping mechanisms to mask their ADHD traits, making it harder to recognize and diagnose. It's crucial to advocate for ourselves, provide a thorough account of our experiences, and seek healthcare providers who understand the nuances of ADHD in women.

Once diagnosed, seeking support and treatment is vital for managing ADHD effectively. Treatment options may include medication, therapy, coaching, and lifestyle adjustments. Collaborating with healthcare professionals and creating a personalized treatment plan tailored to your specific needs can empower you to thrive and embrace your journey with ADHD.

EMBRACING YOUR ADHD IDENTITY

SHIFTING YOUR PERSPECTIVE AND GAINING ACCEPTANCE

Embracing your ADHD as part of your unique identity involves shifting your perspective and reframing the way you perceive your life as a person with ADHD. Instead of viewing ADHD solely as a deficit or a limitation, recognize the strengths and positive aspects that come with it. Embracing your ADHD begins with self-acceptance and understanding that your neurodivergent qualities contribute to your individuality.

EMBRACING STRENGTHS AND UNLEASHING POTENTIAL

ADHD brings a range of strengths, such as creativity, hyperfocus, and the ability to think outside the box. By acknowledging and embracing these strengths, you can leverage them to your advantage. Recognize your unique perspectives and abilities, and find ways to channel them into your personal and professional pursuits to unlock your full potential.

NAVIGATING CHALLENGES WITH RESILIENCE

While embracing your ADHD identity, it's important to acknowledge and navigate the challenges that may arise. Develop resilience by cultivating coping strategies, seeking support from loved ones or support groups, and prioritizing self-care. Embrace the setbacks as opportunities for growth, learning, and developing resilience.

AUTHENTICITY AND SELF-COMPASSION

Embracing your ADHD identity involves being

authentic and true to yourself. Celebrate your uniqueness, and let go of the need to conform to societal expectations or mask your true self. Practice self-compassion by treating yourself with kindness, understanding, and forgiveness. Embrace your imperfections and honor your journey, allowing yourself to grow and flourish as the gifted individual you are.

EMBRACING A TRANSFORMED JOURNEY

EMPOWERMENT THROUGH SELF-UNDERSTANDING

Self-understanding is an essential tool that empowers you to navigate the complexities of life as a woman with ADHD. It allows you to recognize your strengths, manage challenges effectively, and make informed decisions about treatment options, accommodations, and self-care practices. Embrace the knowledge and insight gained through self-understanding as a source of empowerment.

Fostering Growth and Personal Development

Self-understanding opens the door to personal growth and development. By knowing your unique strengths, weaknesses, and triggers, you can focus on personal development strategies that enhance your overall well-being. This may involve cultivating self-care routines, honing time management skills, developing coping mechanisms, or seeking addition education and skills enhancement.

Building Meaningful Connections

Self-understanding can also facilitate the building of meaningful connections and relationships. As you embrace your ADHD identity and develop a deeper understanding of yourself, you can better communicate your needs, establish healthy boundaries, and foster connections with individuals who appreciate and support you. Seek out communities and support networks where you can share experiences, gain insights, and forge lasting relationships with like-minded individuals.

Embracing your ADHD identity and cultivating self-understanding transforms your journey from struggle to growth, acceptance, and empowerment. Embrace the uniqueness of your neurodivergent mind and recognize the vast potential that lies within you. Your self-understanding journey is ongoing, and with each step, you'll continue to evolve, learn, and embrace the radiance of your true self.

CHAPTER 6: UNLEASHING YOUR SUPERPOWERS: TREATMENT AND STRATEGIES

Living with ADHD is like possessing a set of superpowers you have yet to fully understand or control. They can sometimes cause chaos but, when harnessed correctly, can also lead to extraordinary capabilities. This chapter is dedicated to exploring treatments and strategies that can help you unleash these superpowers and thrive with ADHD.

Medical treatments for ADHD have evolved significantly over the years. Stimulant medications such as amphetamine (Adderall) and methylphenidate (Ritalin) have been extensively used and researched.

They work by increasing the levels of certain chemicals in the brain, thereby improving symptoms like inattention, hyperactivity, and impulsivity.

Non-stimulant medications like atomoxetine (Strattera) and guanfacine (Intuniv) are also used, especially for those who don't respond to or can't tolerate stimulants. These medications work differently than stimulants and may have fewer side effects. However, it's essential to remember that medications, while often effective, aren't a one-size-fits-all solution. Each individual responds differently to different medications, and it might take some trial and error to find the most suitable option.

In addition to medications, psychotherapy can also be crucial in treating ADHD. Cognitive-behavioral therapy (CBT), in particular, has shown promising results. CBT focuses on changing thought patterns and behaviors that lead to difficulties. It can help you manage symptoms, cope with challenges, and improve your quality of life.

Beyond the realm of traditional therapies and medications, there exist alternative approaches that can significantly complement ADHD treatment. Mindfulness, a practice rooted in Buddhist meditation, has gained popularity in recent years. It involves paying attention to the present moment without judgment. For those with ADHD, practicing mindfulness can improve attention, reduce stress, and promote emotional regulation.

There are various ways to practice mindfulness, ranging from formal meditation practices like sitting meditation or yoga to informal practices like mindful walking or eating. The key is to find an approach that suits your lifestyle and preferences. You can start with just a few minutes a day and gradually increase the duration as your capacity for mindfulness grows.

Additionally, neurofeedback, a type of biofeedback, has shown promise in treating ADHD. It involves using real-time displays of brain activity—most commonly electroencephalography (EEG)—to teach self-regulation of brain function. While more research is needed to fully establish its effectiveness, some studies suggest that it can improve symptoms of ADHD.

While medical treatments and alternative therapies

can significantly help manage ADHD symptoms, certain lifestyle adjustments can also make a world of difference. Simple changes in diet, exercise, and sleep habits can improve focus and reduce hyperactivity and impulsivity.

For example, diet plays a vital role in managing ADHD. While there's no specific "ADHD diet," following some general guidelines can help improve symptoms. A balanced diet rich in fruits, vegetables, lean proteins, and whole grains can contribute to overall brain health. Omega-3 fatty acids—found in fish, walnuts, and flaxseed—are particularly beneficial and essential for brain function.

While sugar doesn't cause ADHD as was once thought, some people find that limiting sugar and refined carbohydrates helps to reduce hyperactivity and improve concentration. Likewise, some people with ADHD have food sensitivities that may exacerbate symptoms. Keeping a food diary can help identify any links between diet and symptoms.

Exercise is another critical factor in managing ADHD. Regular physical activity can increase the amount of dopamine, norepinephrine, and serotonin in the brain, all of which affect focus and attention. In this way, exercise works in much the same way as ADHD medications like Ritalin and Adderall.

Sleep, too, is fundamental in managing ADHD symptoms. People with ADHD often have disrupted sleep, but a regular sleep routine can help. This includes a consistent bedtime and wake-up time, a cool and dark sleep environment, and a relaxing bedtime routine. Avoiding screens before bed can also improve sleep quality.

A critical aspect of ADHD treatment involves creating a personalized treatment plan for your unique needs and lifestyle. This plan would involve a combination of medical treatments, alternative therapies, and lifestyle changes. It would also incorporate strategies to address specific challenges associated with ADHD, such as time management, organization, and emotional regulation skills.

When creating a personalized treatment plan, working collaboratively with your healthcare provider is essential. Be open about your symptoms, concerns, and goals. Consider all available options, weighing the pros and cons of each. Remember, what works for one person might not work for another, so you may have to try different approaches to find what works best for you.

Furthermore, your personalized plan should be flexible and adaptable. It should evolve as your needs and circumstances change. Regular check-ins with your healthcare provider can help assess the effectiveness of your plan and make necessary adjustments.

It's also essential to involve your support network in your treatment plan. This could include family members, friends, a support group, or an ADHD coach. They can provide emotional support, help you stay accountable, and offer practical assistance.

Moreover, consider incorporating self-care into your treatment plan. Self-care doesn't mean pampering yourself. It's about activities that nourish your physical, emotional, and mental well-being. For someone with ADHD, self-care might mean learning time-management strategies, organization tools, and mindfulness practices or pursuing a hobby that engages your hyperfocus in a positive way.

Lastly, remember that treatment isn't about repairing something that's defective but unleashing your superpowers and using them to create a fulfilling, empowered life.

In the upcoming chapters, we'll discuss life skills and coping mechanisms that can help you thrive with ADHD. We'll also explore the impact of ADHD on relationships and ways to flourish in them. Further, we'll look at strategies to succeed in the workplace and the importance of self-care in managing ADHD.

With the right treatment plan and strategies, you can harness your ADHD superpowers and thrive in all areas of life.

A Short Message from the Author

Hi, are you enjoying the book thus far? I'd love to hear your thoughts! Many readers do not know how hard reviews are to come by, and how much they help an author.

I would be incredibly thankful if you could take just 60 seconds to write a brief review, even if it's just a few sentences!

Thank you for taking the time to share your thoughts!

CHAPTER 7: RHYTHM OF RESILIENCE: LIFE SKILLS AND COPING MECHANISMS

Embracing ADHD is like learning to dance with a vibrant, energetic, and unpredictable partner. It requires a unique set of life skills and coping mechanisms to navigate the complexities and challenges it presents. In this chapter, we'll explore strategies to manage time effectively, regulate emotions, organize your environment, and handle stress to enable you to dance gracefully with your ADHD.

Time Management

Time management is often a significant challenge for those with ADHD. Working with time can seem elusive, making it difficult to plan, prioritize tasks, and adhere to deadlines. However, certain strategies can help you manage time more effectively.

One of these strategies is time blocking, which involves dividing your day into chunks of time dedicated to specific tasks. This gives structure to your day and ensures that you set aside time for all critical activities, including work, leisure, and self-care.

Another strategy is using timers and alarms. These can serve as reminders for starting or ending tasks, taking breaks, and transitioning between activities. For instance, the Pomodoro Technique, in which you work for 25 minutes and then take a five-minute break, can be particularly helpful for maintaining focus and productivity.

It's also crucial to learn to prioritize tasks. Not all tasks are created equal, and it's easy to get overwhelmed if you try to do everything simultaneously. A helpful tool for prioritization is the Eisenhower Matrix, which divides tasks into four categories: urgent and important, important but not urgent, urgent but not important, and not urgent or important. This can help you focus on what truly matters, reducing stress and improving productivity.

EMOTIONAL SELF-REGULATION

Along with time management, emotional self-regulation is another critical area for those with ADHD. ADHD can often lead to intense emotions, difficulty managing those emotions, and impulsive reactions. This can impact various aspects of life, from relationships to work to self-esteem.

Mindfulness is a particularly powerful tool for emotional self-regulation. Mindfulness focuses on paying attention to each moment and your emotional response to what's going on in that moment without judging your reaction. This practice can help you become more aware of your emotions as they arise, allowing you to respond to them consciously rather than reacting impulsively. Simple mindfulness exercises such as focused breathing or body scan meditations can be incorporated into your daily routine.

Another important strategy in regulating emotions is developing a "feelings vocabulary." Being able to name your emotions can help you understand and manage them better. When experiencing a strong emotion, take a moment to identify it. Is it anger? Frustration? Anxiety? Sadness? The simple act of naming the emotion can help you feel more in control.

Creating a self-soothing toolkit can also be helpful. This could include activities that calm you down, comfort items, inspiring quotes, reminders of past successes, or anything else that helps you cope with intense emotions. When you feel overwhelmed, you can turn to your toolkit for support.

Furthermore, consider seeking support from a therapist or coach who specializes in ADHD. They can provide valuable tools and techniques for emotional self-regulation and offer a safe space to explore and process emotions.

ORGANIZATION

Organization is another area where individuals with ADHD often struggle. Cluttered environments can be overwhelming and distracting, making it difficult to focus on and complete tasks. However, you can improve your organizational skills and create an ADHD-friendly environment with a few practical tools and strategies.

Start with simplifying your work and living spaces. The less clutter there is, the less there is to distract you. Regularly declutter your spaces, getting rid of anything you don't need or love.

Next, create designated places for your belongings. "A place for everything, and everything in its place" should be your mantra. This way, you'll know exactly where to find what you need when you need it.

Also, consider using organizing tools that cater to your visual nature. People with ADHD are often visual thinkers, so 'out of sight' often means 'out of mind.' Transparent storage containers, open shelves, and color-coded systems can be extremely helpful.

Don't forget to organize your digital spaces, too. Use digital tools like apps for to-do lists, calendars, and reminders. Regularly declutter your digital files and emails, and organize them into clearly labeled folders.

Lastly, be patient with yourself. Developing organizational skills takes time and practice. Celebrate small victories and progress, and don't beat yourself up if things don't always go as planned.

STRESS MANAGEMENT

Stress management is another vital coping mechanism for those with ADHD. Chronic stress can exacerbate ADHD symptoms and negatively impact your overall health and well-being. Therefore, it's essential to develop strategies to handle stress effectively.

One of the most effective stress-management techniques is regular physical activity. Exercise increases the production of endorphins, your body's natural mood elevators, and can also help improve focus, memory, and sleep, all of which are often

84

problematic for people with ADHD. Find a form of exercise you enjoy, and incorporate it into your daily routine.

Mindfulness and relaxation techniques can also help manage stress. Techniques like deep breathing, progressive muscle relaxation, yoga, and meditation can calm the mind and body, reducing stress and increasing feelings of well-being.

In addition, maintaining a balanced diet can help manage stress. Certain foods can exacerbate stress and ADHD symptoms, while others can help manage them. A diet rich in fruits, vegetables, whole grains, lean proteins, and omega-3 fatty acids can help improve mood, increase energy levels, and stabilize blood sugar, reducing stress and improving ADHD symptoms.

Finally, don't hesitate to seek professional help if you're feeling overwhelmed by stress. Therapists and coaches can provide valuable tools and techniques for stress management, and support groups can offer a safe space to share experiences and coping strategies.

CHAPTER 8: FLOURISHING IN THE GARDEN OF RELATIONSHIPS

ADHD, like the ebb and flow of life's currents, influences and is influenced by the relationships we maintain. The relationships we share with our loved ones are akin to a garden—they require care, attention, and an abundance of love to flourish. In this chapter, we'll learn how to navigate various types of relationships when ADHD is part of the equation.

Starting with personal relationships, which form the core of our social existence, we find that the interplay of ADHD symptoms can sometimes lead to a complex maze of emotions. The inherent challenges posed by ADHD may often strain relationships with family members, close friends, and confidants. Misunderstandings may arise due to perceived inattention or forgetfulness, frustration might build up due to impulsivity, and conflicts may erupt due to difficulty in managing emotions or inconsistency in task execution.

However, it's important to remember that while ADHD might influence these relationships, it doesn't define them. Just as a garden has a variety of flora, our relationships are multifaceted and influenced by a multitude of factors. Once we have an understanding of how ADHD affects us, with a few practical strategies and good communication skills, it's indeed possible for our relationships to not just survive but thrive.

Understanding is the foundation of any relationship. It's crucial for both parties in a relationship—you and your loved one—to understand what ADHD is, how it manifests, and how it affects daily life. This understanding can foster empathy, patience, and effective support. Misconceptions can be cleared, and judgments can be replaced with acceptance.

Communication—the conduit for expressing feelings,

thoughts, needs, and aspirations—is integral to any relationship. For women with ADHD, open and honest communication can help mitigate many potential issues. It allows you to explain your experiences, share your challenges, and express your needs. It also provides an avenue for your loved ones to share their feelings, concerns, and suggestions.

Practical strategies—like calendars or reminders—can be beneficial in managing ADHD symptoms that might impact relationships. For instance, if forgetfulness often leads to missed appointments or unfulfilled promises, setting reminders can help. If impulsivity leads to hasty decisions or actions that impact loved ones, strategies like pausing before responding or decision-making can be helpful.

Next, let's delve into the realm of friendships. Friendships, like beautiful blossoms in a garden, add color, fragrance, and diversity to our lives. Friends provide companionship, mutual support, shared joy, and a sense of belonging. However, managing friendships while dealing with ADHD can sometimes be challenging.

ADHD might lead to difficulty maintaining consistent contact, remembering important dates or details, or managing social commitments. Also, the ups and downs of emotions or struggles with self-image can sometimes make it challenging to forge and maintain friendships. However, the innate creativity, spontaneity, enthusiasm, and resilience of women with ADHD can also make their friendships deep and fulfilling.

As with any personal relationship, understanding, communication, and empathy are vital in managing friendships. It might be helpful to share about your ADHD with your close friends so that they can understand and support you better. Open communication about what you find challenging and how they can help can strengthen the friendship.

Practical strategies can include setting reminders for important dates or commitments, planning ahead for social engagements, or having regular "catch-up" times to maintain contact. Remember, each friendship is unique, and what works best would depend on the dynamics of the particular friendship.

With their added layer of intimacy and commitment, romantic relationships can be a roller-coaster ride for women with ADHD. The intense emotions, the yearning for connection, the fear of rejection, or the struggle with self-image can sometimes be overwhelming. At the same time, the spontaneity, passion, creativity, and resilience that often accompany ADHD can make these relationships deeply fulfilling and exciting.

Understanding your partner's perspective, communicating openly, setting realistic expectations, and working as a team can help you navigate the challenges. For instance, if inattention leads to your partner feeling ignored, it's essential that they understand this is a symptom of ADHD and not a reflection of your love or commitment. If impulsivity leads to conflicts, strategies like taking a timeout during heated moments can help.

Setting boundaries is a vital part of any relationship, but it can be particularly crucial for women with ADHD. Boundaries define the emotional and physical space between you and another person. They express your needs, expectations, and what you consider acceptable behavior. However, setting and maintaining boundaries can sometimes be challenging due to the inherent traits of ADHD, such as impulsivity, desire for immediate reward, or fear of disapproval.

It's essential to remember that setting boundaries isn't about controlling others but about taking care of yourself. Healthy boundaries can help reduce stress, avoid resentment, and promote mutual respect. They can also help manage ADHD symptoms. For instance, if you're easily overwhelmed, setting a boundary about needing quiet time can be beneficial.

In setting boundaries, it's important to be clear, assertive, and consistent. It's also vital to respect others' boundaries. Remember, boundaries aren't rigid walls but flexible lines that can be adjusted in response to changes in the relationship.

As we wrap up this chapter, remember that relationships, like gardens, flourish best with care, patience, and time. ADHD might pose challenges, but it also brings unique strengths. You can nurture your relationships to thrive beautifully with understanding, good communication, effective strategies, and clear boundaries. Reach out for support when needed, learn from shared experiences, and believe in your innate capacity to build and maintain fulfilling relationships.

CHAPTER 9: THE SYMPHONY OF SUCCESS: THRIVING IN THE WORKPLACE

As the lights dim and the curtain rises, we find ourselves in the professional world—a symphony of interlinked tasks, projects, and people, each playing their part to create a harmonious melody. For women with ADHD, this environment can sometimes feel like a stormy sea, filled with distractions, demands, and social intricacies that challenge their unique minds. However, as with any symphony, there's beauty in this complexity—a dance of strengths and challenges that can turn into a powerful, vibrant expression of success when navigated with understanding, creativity, and resilience.

Let's start by exploring the hidden strengths of ADHD in the professional world. ADHD, despite its challenges, often comes with a set of unique skills and abilities that can be especially beneficial in the workplace. This chapter is dedicated to uncovering these skills, understanding how they work, and learning how to leverage them to create a fulfilling professional life.

Many women with ADHD are blessed with a creative, alternative thinking style that can generate innovative ideas and solutions. This creativity can breathe life into projects, lead to inspired problem-solving approaches, and bring a fresh perspective to team discussions.

Additionally, women with ADHD often have the ability to hyperfocus. When channeled into work tasks, this trait can lead to periods of exceptional productivity and achievement.

Lastly, the resilience of living with ADHD can be a powerful asset in the workplace. Women with ADHD face daily challenges that require tenacity, adaptability, and determination—skills that are essential in navigating the trials and tribulations of professional life.

The other side of the coin is that women with ADHD may face challenges at work that their colleagues don't. Acknowledging these not as shortcomings but as aspects requiring extra attention and support is critical. My symphony analogy is about tuning the instruments, adjusting the rhythm, and mastering the pace to allow the music to flow seamlessly.

Common challenges may include staying organized amidst multiple tasks and projects, managing time effectively, maintaining focus in potentially distracting environments, meeting deadlines consistently, or managing complex social interactions. Recognizing these challenges is the first step toward addressing them. Awareness allows us to understand potential obstacles and strategize how to overcome them.

For example, time management is often a challenge for individuals with ADHD. The traditional 9-to-5 work schedule can feel rigid and suffocating, as it doesn't take into account the natural ebb and flow of the ADHD brain. It's not uncommon for women with ADHD to lose track of time, underestimate how long tasks will take, or struggle to prioritize tasks effectively.

However, there are strategies that can help. Breaking tasks into manageable pieces can make them feel less overwhelming and more achievable. Tools like timers, alarms, or digital calendars can help keep track of time and deadlines. Techniques like time blocking or the Pomodoro Technique can provide structure and help manage focus and productivity.

Similarly, staying organized can be a struggle. Juggling multiple tasks, remembering details, or managing paperwork can be overwhelming. However, tools like digital planners, project management apps, or even simple to-do lists can help keep track of tasks, deadlines, and details. Creating systems of organization that work with your unique ADHD brain rather than against it can make a significant difference in managing the workload and reducing stress.

Social interactions in the workplace can also present unique challenges. Sensitivity to criticism, difficulty with small talk, misinterpreting social cues, or feeling overwhelmed by social situations are all challenges that women with ADHD might face. These challenges can impact relationships with colleagues, managers, or clients and can sometimes lead to feelings of isolation or misunderstanding.

However, these social challenges can be navigated successfully with self-awareness, self-acceptance, and a toolkit of coping strategies. Open communication is vital—whether this be explaining your ADHD to colleagues to foster understanding, seeking feedback on the clarity of your communication, or advocating for your needs when necessary. Skills such as active listening, empathy, and assertiveness can also be learned and improved over time.

The workplace is inherently a source of stress with its high demands, tight deadlines, and fast pace. For women with ADHD, this can sometimes exacerbate symptoms or lead to feelings of overwhelm. It's crucial to recognize when you're feeling stressed, take steps to manage this stress, and seek support when needed. Techniques such as mindfulness, deep breathing, or short breaks to move or stretch can help manage stress.

Additionally, recognizing when you need to step back and take care of your mental health is vital. This might mean taking a mental health day, delegating tasks when possible, or seeking support from a counselor or therapist. Remember, taking care of your mental health isn't a sign of weakness but a strength. It's an essential part of ensuring that you can continue to contribute to the workplace in a healthy and sustainable way.

Now that we understand some of the challenges in the workplace for women with ADHD and are aware of possible coping strategies, let's turn our attention to self-advocacy. Advocacy in the workplace is about standing up for your rights, communicating your needs, and creating an environment that supports your success. For women with ADHD, this can mean a variety of things.

Firstly, it might involve disclosing to the appropriate people at your work that you have a diagnosis of ADHD. This is a personal decision and one that requires careful consideration. If you choose to disclose, it can open the door for requesting accommodations, fostering understanding, and advocating for changes that support your productivity and well-being.

Secondly, self-advocacy can mean requesting reasonable accommodations. These accommodations could include changes to your work environment, schedule, or tasks that help mitigate the impact of ADHD on your work performance. For example, you might request a quieter workspace to reduce distractions, flexibility in your work hours to accommodate your natural productivity rhythms, or the use of assistive technology to help with organization and time management.

Lastly, self-advocacy can involve creating boundaries and managing expectations. This might mean saying no to extra work when you're already overloaded, setting clear expectations about your availability, or negotiating more manageable deadlines.

Self-advocacy isn't about asking for special treatment but ensuring that you have the tools and support you need to do your job to the best of your ability. It's about contributing to the symphony of the workplace in a way that your unique talents shine brightly.

Amidst the challenges, let's remember that many women with ADHD don't just survive in the workplace but excel in high positions. They're CEOs, artists, academics, entrepreneurs, healthcare professionals, and so much more. They bring their unique strengths to their work and make significant contributions in their fields.

To illustrate this, let's explore some real-life stories of women who've harnessed their ADHD to achieve professional success. Liz is a successful entrepreneur who runs her own marketing firm. Liz has always had a creative mind, full of innovative ideas. However, she struggled with organization, often feeling overwhelmed by the multiple tasks and deadlines associated with running a business.

Recognizing this, Liz sought support from an ADHD coach who helped her develop systems and strategies to manage her workflow. She started using a digital planner to keep track of tasks and deadlines and introduced regular team meetings to delegate tasks effectively. She also changed her work environment to create a quiet, clutter-free space that helped her focus. Today, Liz's company is thriving, and she credits her success to her creative thinking—a trait she attributes to her ADHD—and the coping strategies she's developed.

You may remember Priya from Chapter 2. She's a university professor who's published numerous research papers in her field. Priya's ADHD makes her a non-linear thinker, able to make connections between ideas that others often miss. However, she struggled with maintaining focus during long hours of research and writing.

Priya began using the Pomodoro Technique to address this, working for focused bursts of time with regular breaks in between. She also began to use speech-to-text software to capture her ideas quickly when she was in a state of hyperfocus. Today, Priya is recognized as a leader in her field, and she believes that her unique perspective—contributed by her ADHD—is a key factor in her success.

These stories illustrate that while ADHD can present challenges, it also brings strengths that can contribute to professional success. Creative thinking, the ability to hyperfocus, resilience, and a unique perspective are all common attributes associated with ADHD that can be harnessed to succeed in the workplace.

However, it's important to note that success doesn't always look like high-profile careers or external achievements. Success can also mean finding work that you love, work that aligns with your values, or work that allows you to balance your professional and personal life in a way that supports your well-being. It's about finding your unique path—your own symphony of success.

In conclusion, thriving in the workplace as a woman with ADHD involves understanding and managing your symptoms, advocating for your needs, and leveraging your unique strengths. It's about creating an environment where you can shine brightly—not to compensate for your ADHD but to take advantage of it.

The path might not always be smooth. There might be days of self-doubt, challenges that seem insurmountable, or setbacks that knock you off course. But remember, just as a symphony requires both soft, slow movements and fast, intense ones to create a beautiful piece of music, so does your journey with ADHD. It's the challenges, victories, setbacks, and progress that shape you, strengthen you, and enable you to create your own unique symphony of success.

And, with that, we end Chapter 9, hopeful that you're now equipped with a better understanding of how to navigate and thrive in the workplace as a woman with ADHD. In the next chapter, we'll explore the importance of self-care, providing you with practical strategies to nurture your physical, emotional, and mental health.

Chapter 10: Your Sanctuary of Self-Care: Nourishing the Mind, Body, and Soul

Self-care is a term we often hear today, yet it remains a concept that's frequently misunderstood. We see it on social media, where influencers encourage us to treat ourselves to a day at the spa or a shopping spree. We hear it in conversation when we're encouraged to "take time for ourselves." But what does self-care truly mean, and why is it particularly crucial for women with ADHD?

In essence, self-care means nurturing our physical, emotional, and mental well-being. It's about creating a sanctuary within ourselves where we can retreat, rejuvenate, and recharge. For women with ADHD, this sanctuary becomes even more important due to the unique challenges associated with the condition.

Living with ADHD often feels like being in a constant state of overstimulation. Your thoughts may run a mile a minute, making it difficult to focus on a single task. The world around you might seem too loud, too bright, too busy. It can be easy to get overwhelmed, leading to heightened stress levels and, in some cases, burnout.

Moreover, women with ADHD often face additional societal pressures. Many women are expected to take on multiple roles—as a professional, a caregiver, a partner, and a parent. These roles can come with a plethora of responsibilities, leaving little time for rest and relaxation. When you add ADHD into the mix, the stress can intensify, making self-care not just important but essential.

Remember, self-care isn't about being selfish or indulgent. It's about recognizing that you, too, deserve care and attention. It's about acknowledging that, for you to be of the most benefit to yourself and others, you need to tend to your own needs. It's about transforming self-care from an occasional treat into a non-negotiable part of your daily routine.

So, let's discover what self-care means for you. Let's create a sanctuary where you can retreat when the world becomes too overwhelming. Let's learn how to nurture yourself as someone who experiences both the challenges and blessings of ADHD.

To create a self-care routine that truly meets your needs as a woman with ADHD, it's essential to start by understanding what self-care means to you personally. Self-care is a highly individualized practice, as everyone has unique preferences, interests, and needs. What brings you joy, relaxation, and a sense of well-being might differ from what works for someone else. Listening to your intuition and exploring activities that resonate with you is essential.

Physical self-care involves caring for your body, ensuring it receives the nourishment, movement, and rest it needs. For women with ADHD, engaging in regular exercise can have profound benefits. Exercise has been shown to improve focus, attention, and overall cognitive function. Finding physical activities align with your well-being or that would overburden your schedule. Setting boundaries protects your time and energy and allows you to make space for self-care practices that nourish and rejuvenate you.

Incorporating self-care into your schedule may require some planning and intentionality. Consider blocking off specific time slots dedicated to self-care activities just as you would for a work meeting or appointment. Treat these time blocks as sacred and non-negotiable, recognizing that taking care of yourself is a priority.

Additionally, remember that self-care doesn't have to be elaborate or time-consuming. It can be as simple as taking a few minutes each day to engage in deep breathing exercises, enjoy a cup of tea, go for a walk in Nature, or indulge in a relaxing bath. Find activities that bring you joy, peace, and a sense of grounding, and incorporate them into your daily routine.

Practicing self-care also means recognizing when you need professional help. If you find that your ADHD symptoms are significantly impacting your daily life, or you're struggling with mental health concerns, seeking the guidance of a healthcare professional such as a therapist or psychiatrist can be beneficial. They can provide personalized strategies, treatment options, and support to navigate the challenges you may face.

Lastly, remember that self-care is an ongoing process. As you evolve and grow, your self-care needs may change. It's important to regularly check in with yourself, reassess your self-care routine, and adjust as needed. Be open to exploring new activities, techniques, or approaches that resonate with your current needs and desires.

In conclusion, creating a self-care sanctuary as a woman with ADHD involves nurturing your physical, emotional, and mental well-being. It requires prioritizing yourself, setting boundaries, and engaging in activities that bring you joy, relaxation, and a sense of balance. Remember that self-care isn't a luxury but an essential practice that allows you to thrive and show up as your best self in all areas of your life.

resilience and growth.

Additionally, social media platforms can be valuable tools for sharing your experiences on a larger scale. Create a blog, Instagram account, or YouTube channel dedicated to raising awareness about ADHD and empowering women. Use these platforms to share educational content, personal stories, and resources that can support and uplift others in the ADHD community.

Remember, sharing your experiences is a personal choice. It's important to be aware of and respect your own boundaries and only share what feels comfortable for you. By sharing authentically and responsibly, you can make a meaningful impact and help create a more understanding and inclusive world for women with ADHD.

ADVOCACY ON A LARGER SCALE

Advocacy doesn't stop at sharing your personal experiences. It can also involve advocating for wider societal changes and understanding of ADHD. By raising your voice and advocating on a larger scale, you can contribute to the well-being and empowerment of all women with ADHD.

One effective way to do this is by getting involved in ADHD advocacy organizations and initiatives. These organizations work tirelessly to promote ADHD awareness, provide resources and support, and advocate for policy changes. Consider joining a local or national ADHD advocacy group, attending conferences or events, and volunteering your time to support their efforts. Together, we can amplify our voices and bring about positive change.

Educating others about ADHD is another crucial aspect of advocacy. Use your knowledge and experiences to raise awareness and challenge misconceptions. Offer educational presentations at schools, workplaces, or community events to increase understanding and promote empathy. By sharing accurate information and dispelling myths, you can be an ambassador for your sisters with ADHD.

Moreover, advocacy involves speaking up for yourself in various settings, including the workplace, educational institutions, and healthcare systems. Learn about your rights, legal protections, and available accommodations. Be prepared to communicate your needs clearly and assertively, and don't hesitate to ask for reasonable accommodations that can help level the playing field and support your success.

LEADING BY EXAMPLE

Throughout history, many remarkable women with ADHD have emerged as strong advocates for themselves and others. Their stories inspire us and remind us of the power of perseverance, resilience, and the ability to create positive change. Here are a few of these strong women and their inspiring stories:

1. Temple Grandin: Temple Grandin is a renowned author, speaker, and autism advocate. She's also spoken openly about her ADHD diagnosis and how it's influenced her life. Despite facing numerous challenges, Temple has become a leading advocate for individuals with autism and ADHD by using

her unique perspective and experiences to educate others and promote understanding.

2. Jessica McCabe: Jessica McCabe is the creator of the popular YouTube channel, "How to ADHD," where she shares her experiences with ADHD and provides valuable insights and strategies for managing symptoms. Through her engaging videos, Jessica has become a beacon of hope and inspiration for thousands of individuals with ADHD.

3. Sari Solden: Sari Solden is a psychotherapist, author, and pioneer in the field of women with ADHD. She's dedicated her career to advocating for women with ADHD, conducting workshops, and providing guidance to help them better understand their strengths and challenges. Her work has had a profound impact on empowering women with ADHD to embrace their uniqueness and thrive.

These women, among many others, serve as role models for empowerment and advocacy. Their stories remind us that we have the power to create change— not just in our own lives but also in the lives of others facing similar challenges. By sharing our stories, supporting one another, and advocating for understanding and acceptance, we can create a world where women with ADHD can thrive.

TAKING ACTION

Now that you understand the importance of advocacy and have heard the inspiring stories of women who've become advocates for themselves and others, it's time to take action in your own life. Here are some practical steps you can take to further empower yourself and advocate for the ADHD community:

1. Educate yourself: Expand your knowledge about ADHD by reading books, articles, and research papers. Stay updated on the latest advancements in ADHD treatment and support. The more you understand about ADHD, the better equipped you'll be to advocate for yourself and educate others.

2. Seek support: Build a support network by connecting with other women with ADHD. Join support groups, both online and in-

person, where you can share experiences, learn from others, and gain valuable insights. Surrounding yourself with like-minded individuals can provide a sense of validation and strength.

3. Speak up: Don't be afraid to share your experiences and advocate for your needs. Whether in personal relationships, the workplace, or educational settings, assertively communicate your challenges and views. Be confident in expressing your unique strengths and contributions.

4. Share your story: Consider sharing your journey with ADHD through writing, speaking engagements, or social media. Your story has the power to inspire and empower others. Speaking openly about your experiences can challenge stereotypes, break down stigmas, and promote understanding.

5. Get involved: Engage in advocacy efforts by joining ADHD organizations, attending events, or participating in awareness campaigns. Volunteer your time, share resources, and contribute your unique perspectives and

talents to make a difference in the ADHD community.

Remember, advocacy isn't a one-time action but an ongoing journey. As you continue to empower yourself and advocate for others, you're making a positive impact and lighting the way for women with ADHD to thrive.

CONCLUSION

"We do not need magic to transform our world. We carry all of the power we need inside ourselves already." - J.K. Rowling

As we come to the end of this empowering journey, it's time to reflect on the lessons learned, the growth experienced, and the vast potential that lies within each and every woman with ADHD. Throughout this book, we investigated the many challenging and inspiring aspects of ADHD, explored its impact on women's lives, and discovered strategies for empowerment, self-care, and advocacy. Now, in this concluding chapter, let's take a moment to celebrate how far you've come, embrace the radiant journey that lies ahead, and offer final words of encouragement to uplift your spirit.

Reflecting on our journey together, we can see the transformative power of understanding, compassion, and self-discovery. You embarked on this path with an open mind and an eagerness to explore the unique challenges and strengths of women with ADHD. You've gained insights into the complex nature of ADHD, debunked myths and stereotypes, and recognized the immense potential that lies within you.

Throughout these chapters, you've discovered the hidden strengths of ADHD and have gained new insights into the unique attributes often found in individuals with ADHD. You've explored the female experience of ADHD, navigating the challenges specific to women and discovering strategies for overcoming hurdles. You've delved into the power of community and found solace in the shared journey of women with ADHD. You've unraveled the gift of self-understanding, recognizing the significance of embracing your ADHD as part of your unique identity.

You've explored treatment options, coping mechanisms, and life skills to unleash your superpowers and thrive in various aspects of life. You've learned the art of self-care, nurturing your physical, emotional, and mental well-being. You've embraced your role as an advocate, empowering yourself and lighting the way for others.

Embracing your ADHD is a powerful step toward self-acceptance and personal growth. As you journeyed through this book, you've learned that ADHD isn't a flaw or a limitation but a unique part of your identity. It brings a set of strengths such as creativity, intuition, and a unique perspective on the world. By embracing your ADHD, you can harness these strengths to achieve personal and professional success.

You've learned that embracing your ADHD doesn't mean ignoring its challenges. It means acknowledging them, seeking needed support, and developing strategies to manage them effectively. It means understanding that your journey may be different from others, and that's perfectly okay. Embracing your ADHD is about cultivating self-compassion, celebrating your achievements, and accepting yourself fully.

As you continue your journey, you now know the importance of surrounding yourself with a supportive network of individuals who understand and uplift you and seeking out communities, support groups, and connections with like-minded individuals who share similar experiences. Together, you can provide encouragement, share insights, and remind one another of the profound strengths that come with ADHD.

As you stand at the culmination of this transformative journey, it's important to look ahead with optimism and anticipation. You've acquired a wealth of knowledge, tools, and strategies to navigate the challenges of ADHD, nurture your well-being, and advocate for yourself and others. Armed with this newfound understanding and empowerment, you can shape a future that's aligned with your special gifts.

In the days and years to come, remember to continue prioritizing self-care. The practices and routines you've established throughout this book are meant to serve as enduring pillars of your well-being. Make a conscious effort to carve out time for activities that bring you joy, peace, and rejuvenation. Whether engaging in hobbies, practicing mindfulness, or connecting with Nature, consistently nurturing your physical, emotional, and mental health will fortify your resilience and equip you to face the challenges that may arise.

Additionally, keep the flame of advocacy burning brightly within you. Your journey has empowered you to become an advocate not just for yourself but for the broader ADHD community. Share your story, raise awareness, and challenge misconceptions whenever and wherever possible. By doing so, you'll continue to make a profound impact, breaking down barriers and fostering understanding and acceptance.

Finally, celebrate your progress and achievements, no matter how small they may seem. Recognize the growth you've undergone throughout this journey, the resilience you've developed, and the unique strengths you possess. Give yourself permission to celebrate your victories and embrace the radiant, limitless potential that lies within you.

As we near the end of this book, I want to offer you some final words of encouragement. Remember that you're not alone on this journey. Countless women with ADHD, like yourself, are navigating the intricacies of life with strength and determination. Reach out to your support network, connect with others who understand, and draw inspiration from their stories.

Embrace the challenges and triumphs that come with ADHD, for they've shaped you into the remarkable woman you are today. Your unique perspective, creativity, and resilience set you apart. Embrace your quirks, your abilities, and the beautiful complexity that makes you who you are.

Know that growth is a continuous process. Be patient with yourself as you navigate the ups and downs of your ADHD journey. Some days may feel more challenging than others, but remember that every step forward, no matter how small, is progress. Be kind to yourself and celebrate each milestone along the way.

Lastly, never underestimate the impact you can make. As you embrace your own empowerment, you become a beacon for others. Share your experiences, offer support and guidance, and advocate for understanding and acceptance. Doing so contributes to a more compassionate and inclusive world for women with ADHD.

The radiant journey ahead is yours to embrace, filled with endless possibilities and opportunities for growth. Trust in your inner strength, believe in your abilities, and continue to nurture your well-being. You can achieve greatness, and your unique journey with ADHD will continue to shape your path in remarkable ways.

As we conclude this transformative journey, I want to express my deepest gratitude for joining me on this exploration of empowerment, self-care, and advocacy for women with ADHD. Your commitment to personal growth and embracing your true potential is truly inspiring.

Remember that this book is just the beginning of your path to empowerment. The insights, strategies, and stories you've encountered within these pages are meant to guide and support you, but the true power lies within you. Carry the wisdom you've gained, and continue to cultivate your self-awareness, self-care practices, and advocacy efforts. Embrace your journey with open arms and an unwavering belief in your ability to thrive.

As you venture forth, challenges will arise, but you have the tools and knowledge to navigate them with grace. Tap into the strengths that come with ADHD, draw upon the support of your community, and never underestimate the power of self-advocacy.

May this journey be a catalyst for positive change in your life and the lives of those around you. Shine your light eagerly, embrace your authenticity, and continue to inspire others through your unique journey with ADHD. Together, we can create a world where women with ADHD are empowered, understood, and celebrated for their remarkable strengths.

With heartfelt gratitude and warm wishes on your continued journey.

ONE MORE THING

If you enjoyed this book and found it helpful, I'd be very grateful if you'd post a short review on Amazon. Your support does make a difference, and I read all the reviews personally so I can get your feedback and make this book even better. I love hearing from my readers, and I'd really appreciate it if you leave your honest feedback.

Thank you for reading!

BONUS CHAPTER

I would like to share a sneak peek into another one of my books that I think you will enjoy. The book is titled "Women with ADHD Falling through the Cracks: Unmasking the Bias and Exploring Why ADD and ADHD Symptoms in Adult Women and Girls Are Misunderstood and Undiagnosed."

Women with attention-deficit/hyperactivity disorder (ADHD) are falling through the cracks, and it's time to talk about it.

ADHD is not just a problem for kids and males. With centuries of cultural stereotypes about women's supposed lack of intellect, women with ADHD are often overlooked and unacknowledged. 50%-75% of ADHD cases in females are missed.

This diagnosis gap happens partly because it's a condition that was traditionally thought to affect mostly men, but also because women tend to have less obvious or socially disruptive symptoms than men. Males tend to be diagnosed more often and sooner because their symptoms are usually more physical and obvious. Inattentive ADHD, the most common ADHD presentation in females, tends to be mental rather than physical. Since many of these symptoms take place inside the mind, they can be easy for parents, patients and mental health professionals to miss.

ADHD is a challenging condition for women and girls. According to the Centers for Disease Control and Prevention, the diagnosis rate among females is 40% lower than males. The symptoms can be different but the consequences are just as serious. Women with ADHD often go undiagnosed or misdiagnosed, which negatively impacts their mental & physical wellbeing and relationships. The good news? ADHD can be managed with medication and coaching. This book introduces ADHD through the lens of women, offers tips for managing daily life, and includes a list of resources for women in particular.

This book will teach you:
- What is ADHD

- How to diagnose ADHD
- ADHD management strategies
- Tips for parents of an ADHD child
- Treatment options of ADHD
- How ADHD symptoms differs in women
- Why ADHD Is Underdiagnosed in Women
- Challenges of women with ADHD

If you are a woman with ADHD, you should know that it is a very treatable condition. As overwhelmed as you may feel, know that you can feel better. There is a lot you can do to regain control of your life, instead of having ADHD control you. It's time to Know Your ADHD and Own Your ADHD!

Enjoy this free chapter!

The majority of research on attention deficit hyperactivity disorder (ADHD) has traditionally focused on males, who were believed to make up 80% of all those with ADHD. Now more and more females are being identified, especially now that we are more aware of the non-hyperactive subtype of ADHD. Girls and women with ADHD struggle with a variety of issues that are different from those faced by males. This book will highlight some of those differences, and we will explore the types of struggles faced by females with ADHD.

ADHD is a neurodevelopmental disorder characterized by impulsive behavior and related symptoms. The disorder is classified into three types: impulsive/hyperactivity, inattention/distractibility, and a combination.

While ADHD is the most common disorder among boys aged four to eleven, only about half as many girls are diagnosed, according to the Australian Institute of Health and Welfare. While women tend to develop ADHD later in life, most symptoms appear in infancy and go undiagnosed, untreated, or are well-masked by social and communication abilities.

According to Mark Bellgrove, a professor of cognitive neuroscience, females with ADHD are more likely than males to abuse substances. He stated, "As a result, we want to catch them sooner and treat them more effectively. However, I believe it is safe to say they are slipping through the cracks."

According to some studies, up to three-quarters of adult women with ADHD are undiagnosed. Many women diagnosed with ADHD as adults reflect on the red flags they ignored as children, such as difficulties in school or difficulties making friends. They wonder how their lives would have changed if their condition had been identified earlier. Coping with symptoms becomes more difficult for those not diagnosed as their responsibilities grow in adulthood.

According to ADHD-specialist psychologist Tamara May, some women receive an ADHD diagnosis after years of struggling with symptoms of "secondary" depression and anxiety due to the problem not being diagnosed. "During adolescence, many women realize they are struggling more than their classmates, but they don't know why," she adds. People underestimate the severity of ADHD and how difficult even the most basic tasks can be. "You're being lazy; you should be able to do better," people around them say. Simply getting up and doing the dishes can be a challenge.

This medical issue is exacerbated by the fact that there are a limited number of psychiatrists who specialize in ADHD, almost all of whom work in the private sector. According to Dr. May, it is extremely rare for someone to be diagnosed in the public hospital system. "Women must first recognize that they are experiencing symptoms of ADHD before consulting with their primary care physician and obtaining a referral to see a private psychiatrist. Waitlists range from three to six months, and some psychiatrists have closed their doors." Some women have reported spending up to $2,000 to get a diagnosis confirmed.

Furthermore, obtaining ADHD medication necessitates a consultation with a psychiatrist. Women who want to change their lives by recognizing and accepting their ADHD must take the initiative. While public awareness of adult ADHD is growing, research biases persist. Women's specific complications such as the effects of pregnancy, menopause, hormones, and the menstrual cycle on ADHD symptoms have received little attention.

Women are just as negatively affected by ADHD as men, if not more so. While most ADHD research has focused on white male participants, some studies have included or focused on the life outcomes of adult female ADHD patients. This book does a detailed analysis and provides helpful solutions.

ADHD is a disorder with a high comorbidity rate. It has been determined that ADHD in a girl or woman increases the likelihood that she will experience trauma at some point in her life. The most common comorbid diagnoses in women are depression, anxiety, and eating disorders. While these diagnoses frequently co-occur, it has been discovered that many women are misdiagnosed with conditions such as anxiety or depression when the underlying issue is ADHD. Unintended pregnancies, marital abuse, and an increased risk of self-harm and suicide are more common in women with ADHD than in the general population. While the literature indicates that living with ADHD hurts both men and women, gender differences among people with ADHD have not been thoroughly investigated. However, this research is necessary because the number of women diagnosed with ADHD has risen in recent years. This is partly due to practitioners' increased awareness that not only can ADHD persist into adulthood, but it is also not a gender-based illness.

Women whose disabilities or struggles may have gone

unnoticed or been misinterpreted during childhood and adolescence struggle to cope with the inevitable increase in adult responsibilities. This trend has been picked up and written about in the popular press. Many doctors and psychiatrists agree that a lack of research is a problem. They believe that advances in this area could reduce stigma and provide greater inclusion for people with ADHD and other illnesses.

Despite the bad press and lack of research, there are success stories. Ms. Josie Bober's is one. Despite consistently high grades, Ms. Bober had been unable to complete any of the university degrees she had begun before her diagnosis. Despite her illness, she recently completed a graphic design degree and is now determined to help others by making universities more welcoming to neurodiverse people. Her alma mater, the University of New South Wales, has even provided her with funding to conduct workshops with students and professors to develop effective strategies. In her interview, she stated, "I was feeling proactive. I believe I reached a point within myself where I felt confident and eager to help others. "Increased ADHD diagnoses among women should improve their overall performance and quality of life. However, a lack of research on women with ADHD may result in gender-specific requirements and overlooked obstacles in this population."

This book offers a comprehensive insight into the identification, treatment, and support for girls and women with ADHD. It is critical to reject the widely held belief that ADHD is a behavioral disorder and concentrate on the more subtle and internalized presentation typical of females. Adopting a lifelong model of care is critical to assist the multiple transitions that females experience concurrently with changes in their clinical presentation and social situations. Treatment with pharmacological and psychological therapies is expected to increase productivity, reduce resource use, and, most importantly, better the long-term outcomes for girls and women.

Understanding ADHD

Attention Deficit Hyperactivity Disorder (ADHD) is a neurological condition that affects a person's thoughts, behaviors, and ability to process information. It mainly affects children and adolescents; however, it may affect adults too. Approximately 11 percent of children between four and seventeen have ADHD, and around four percent of adults in the U.S. suffer from the condition. It's three times more common in boys than girls.

ADHD is classified as a neurodevelopmental disorder, similar to disorders such as autism, and is not a mental illness. Neurodevelopmental conditions arise when the nervous system's development is compromised during the early stages of childhood. This is due to a combination of genetic, neurological, and environmental factors.

ADHD comes in three types: Inattentive, Hyperactive-Impulsive, and Combination. Each type of ADHD is associated with one or more distinguishing features. Individuals with the inattentive form are easily distracted and have difficulty concentrating and organizing their thoughts. Individuals with the hyperactive-impulsive type often fidget when speaking and struggle to stay focused on a job. Finally, those with the combination type of ADHD often interrupt while others are talking, appear not to listen when spoken to, become easily distracted, and are fond of taking risks.

You can only know the type of ADHD you have based on your symptoms. Because everyone is unique, two individuals may have the same symptoms yet interpret them differently. Males and females, for example, often behave differently anyway. Males could be seen as more energetic, whereas girls may be viewed as calmer and more uninterested in risky behavior.

RECENT STUDIES AND STATISTICS

Until recently, ADHD was thought to be a disorder that only affected children. According to the most recent estimates, 9.6 percent of children between the ages of three and 17 have been diagnosed with this issue.

According to novel research published in the *American Journal of Psychiatry*, about 10 percent of persons with ADHD grow out of it. Even if individuals have symptom-free periods, 90 percent will suffer from at least moderate symptoms throughout adulthood. This study's authors considered ADHD an episodic condition with symptoms that vary and change based on life circumstances. Many children with ADHD, for example, may seem to be symptom-free at the age of 18 while still in high school and living at home. When those same teenagers go off to college, their ADHD symptoms may resurface owing to the stress that often comes with a change in environment. Experts have long known that anxiety and lack of sleep may exacerbate ADHD symptoms. These researchers intend to focus their future study on potential causes and supports for patients with ADHD. The results collated from the Multimodal Treatment of Attention

Deficit Hyperactivity Study (MTA), a federally sponsored experiment, are presented in this report. The MTA began in 1998 and followed roughly 600 children from the ages of seven to nine until they reached the age of 25. They lived at eight different locations throughout the nation.

The Centers for Disease Control and Prevention (CDC) conducted a study in 2016. They discovered that around 6.1 million children between the ages of two and 17 (9.4 percent) had been diagnosed with ADHD. The condition has also been identified in 388,000 (2.4 percent) children aged two to five, 2.4 million (9.6 percent) school-aged children aged six to 11 years, and 3.3 million (13.6 percent) teenagers aged 12 to 17 years. Based on their research, the CDC concluded that males are more likely than females to be diagnosed with ADHD. (12.9 percent and 5.6 percent, respectively).

However, new research shows that ADHD affects a more significant percentage of females than is often recognized. Because of how girls' symptoms develop compared to boys', ADHD may be overlooked in females, indicating a general bias in the diagnosing process. According to the DSM-5, ADHD is one of childhood's most frequent neurodevelopmental disorders. While estimates vary, the global incidence of ADHD in adolescents is about 5 percent.

According to a study by the Centers for Disease Control and Prevention (CDC) in 2016, the global prevalence of adult ADHD is predicted to be 2.8 percent. Adult ADHD prevalence estimates in the United States vary. According to one research paper published in 2019, the prevalence of adult ADHD is 0.96 percent, up from 0.43 percent a decade before. Adult ADHD prevalence rates in the United States have previously been estimated to range between 2.5 percent and 4.4 percent, with males being diagnosed at 5.4 percent compared to 3.2 percent for women.

ADHD Brain VS Normal Brain

Researchers discovered that the cerebral cortex, limbic system, and reticulating activating systems in individuals with ADHD are distinct from those of others. These differences explain short attention spans, learning problems, emotional instability, and restlessness. The cerebral cortex is the brain's outermost layer and is responsible for our highest mental abilities like thought, reasoning, and language. It has been shown that patients with ADHD exhibit slower brain wave activity. Through brain imaging studies, researchers were able to identify that the right frontal lobe of those with ADHD is also smaller than the frontal lobe in individuals without ADHD. This part of the brain is responsible for paying attention, focusing, and concentrating. It is in charge of planning, making choices, learning, remembering, and acceptable behavior. The cortex controls impulse and improper behavior by "inhibitory mechanisms" in the cortex.

The limbic system is the region of the brain located just above the brain stem. It is responsible for one's feelings, motivations, and survival instinct. The limbic system also regulates what is recalled and where memories are kept in the brain. The limbic system – consisting of the hypothalamus, amygdala, and hippocampus – helps us respond to emotional stimuli and is responsible for integrating our bodily senses to make sense of what is happening in the world around us, such as temperature changes, body position, and hormone levels. If the limbic system gets overwhelmed or receives excessive information from the body simultaneously, problems can occur.

The reticulating activating system (RAS) is also found near the spinal cord at the base of the brain. It receives information about the world and one's own body through the senses. It activates cerebral cortex neurons which are in charge of circadian rhythms (sleep and wake cycles), central nervous system activity, and attention. When the RAS is underactive, it causes learning, memory, and self-control problems. However, when the RAS is overactive, the individual becomes easily startled, speaks excessively, and becomes anxious and hyperactive. A shutdown of the RAS causes the loss of consciousness or coma.

NEURODIVERSITY

There's a lot of debate over whether ADHD should be classified as a mental illness. Even though some persons with ADHD exhibit mental abnormalities and severe impairment, some experts still do not consider these abnormalities to indicate a disorder. Instead, they consider these anomalies as usual but extreme.

The term "neurodiversity" is used by researchers to characterize normal, hereditary, brain-based behavioral variances. Certain conditions, classified as diseases, show a total and utter departure from normal and healthy functioning (e.g., diabetes). Similarly, certain conditions are not disease states, yet not everyone has them. For instance, pregnancy. In both circumstances, though, it's all or nothing. You can't be a little bit pregnant or diabetic. These conditions either affect you or do not affect you. Consider it as if you were switching on a light. It can only be turned on or off.

However, unlike many biologically-based symptoms, behavioral symptoms may be a question of degree. There are certain behaviors that almost everyone exhibits to some extent (e.g., inattention). Consider it like a dimmer switch with an endless intensity range between on and off. ADHD is similar to a light switch with a light. It's defined by a set of characteristics (inattention, impulsivity, excessive energy, and distraction) that everyone exhibits to varying degrees. As a result, the issue becomes: At what point does it constitute a disorder?

According to the neurodiversity argument, ADHD is not an unnatural condition since a considerable section of the population exhibits ADHD-like behaviors, although to a lesser degree. It's just an extreme case of a standard variety. As previously stated, to add to the confusion, symptoms such as impulsivity and high energy are not exclusive to ADHD. These signs and symptoms may be seen in a variety of illnesses. The fact that ADHD symptoms aren't exclusive to that condition supports the neurodiversity argument that ADHD isn't an actual disorder.

WHAT ARE THE SYMPTOMS OF ADHD?

Adults with ADHD may have difficulty listening carefully, impulsivity, and anxiety. The signs and symptoms might be modest to severe. While some individuals with ADHD have fewer symptoms as they get older, others have significant symptoms that affect their daily routine.

Many adults with ADHD aren't even aware that they have it; all they know is that regular activities are challenging for them. Adults with ADHD may have trouble focusing and prioritizing, leading to missed deadlines and forgotten meetings or social activities. The inability to manage impulses may manifest in various ways, from irritation when standing in a queue or driving in traffic to bouts of depression and angry outbursts.

Impulsivity, difficulty with multitasking, poor planning, poor organizational skills, disorientation, and issues with prioritizing are some of the symptoms of adult ADHD—as well as low tolerance for frustration, regular mood fluctuations, and issues with completing tasks.

Inattentive ADHD

Inattentive ADHD (often called ADD) manifests as forgetfulness, disengagement, or distractibility, and can be mistaken for anxiety or a mood disorder in adults. Those with inattentive ADHD make mistakes because they cannot stay focused, organize tasks or activities, or follow instructions. They often lose things and become easily distracted by certain external stimuli. Here are some symptoms of Inattentive-Type ADHD:

- Often fails to give close attention to details or makes careless mistakes
- Easily distracted
- Often does not seem to listen when spoken to directly
- Often has trouble organizing tasks and activities
- Often avoids, dislikes, or is reluctant to do tasks that require mental effort over a long period
- Often loses things necessary for tasks and activities

- Forgetful
- Ignores tasks they find boring
- Difficulty learning new information
- Frequent "spaciness"
- Daydreams regularly

Co-occurring Conditions with ADHD

Learning disabilities – Learning disabilities make it difficult for a child to master certain skills, such as reading or arithmetic. While ADHD is not a learning disability, it can make it difficult for a child to do well in school. Diagnosing learning disabilities requires assessments such as IQ and academic achievement tests. Such disabilities require educational interventions once identified.

Oppositional defiant disorder or conduct disorder – Up to 35 percent of children with ADHD also have an oppositional defiant disorder or conduct disorder. Children with such disorders tend to lose their cool quickly. In addition, they are defiant and hostile towards authority figures. Children with conduct disorder break rules, destroy things, and often get suspended or expelled from school. Children with co-occurring conduct disorder are at much higher risk of having problems with the law or substance abuse than children with ADHD alone. Studies show that this co-existing condition is more common among children with the mainly hyperactive/impulsive type of ADHD and the combined type of ADHD.

Mood disorders/depression – Approximately 18 percent of children with ADHD also have mood disorders such as depression or bipolar disorder (previously called manic depression). There is often a family history of these types of disorders. Co-existing mood disorders can put children at higher risk for suicide, especially during the teen years. These disorders are more common among children who have the inattentive type of ADHD and the combined type of ADHD.

Anxiety disorders – Anxiety affects about 25 percent of children with ADHD. Children with anxiety disorders have extreme feelings of fear, worry, or panic that make it difficult to function. These disorders can produce physical symptoms such as rapid heartbeat, sweating, diarrhea, and nausea. Different counseling and medications may be needed to treat these co-existing conditions.

Language disorders – Children with ADHD may have difficulty with the way they use language. This is known as a *pragmatic language disorder*. It may not show up on standard language tests. A speech and language specialist can detect this by observing how the child uses language in their daily activities.

164

Diagnosing ADHD

A physical examination, such as a blood test or an X-ray, cannot diagnose ADHD. An assessment technique is used instead by a health professional to diagnose ADHD. Regardless of how ADHD manifests—inattentive, hyperactive-impulsive, or combined—several characteristics must be satisfied before an official diagnosis can be made.

Some of these requirements include:

1. Presence of symptoms before the age of twelve.

2. Observed symptoms should be evident in a variety of circumstances.

3. Observed symptoms have to interfere with or affect one's daily routine.

4. No other mental health disease can explain the symptoms.

A medical interview with a mental health expert qualified to assess and diagnose Attention Deficit Hyperactivity Disorder (ADHD) is used to diagnose the disorder in children and adolescents. Mental health professionals, psychologists, and neurologists that focus on dealing with children and adolescents are the most prevalent practitioners in this field. Neuropsychological testing may help reach a diagnosis, but it is insufficient without a clinical evaluation. Brain imaging techniques such as MRI, CT, and PET scans are not used to diagnose ADHD in children because none of these tools can be used as accurate tools to identify the condition. They may help give the diagnosing professional extra information, but they are not diagnostic on their own.

A child must show at least six ADHD symptoms of inattention, hyperactivity-impulsivity, or both to be diagnosed with ADHD. To establish that a child has ADHD, the symptoms must have been present for at least six months and must have appeared before age seven.

The most common symptoms observed include having trouble keeping attention, listening or following directions, making careless errors, avoiding jobs that demand continuous concentration, being forgetful, becoming sidetracked quickly, and losing things easily.

ADHD in Children

Children with ADHD may have poor self-esteem, strained relationships, and poor academic achievement. Symptoms may reduce as they become older. Some individuals, however, never fully recover from their ADHD symptoms. They can, however, develop effective coping tactics.

Medications and behavioral approaches are often used together in treatment. While medication will not cure ADHD, it may significantly reduce its symptoms. Early detection and treatment may have a significant impact on the person's quality of life.

Inattention and hyperactive-impulsive behavior are two of the most common symptoms of ADHD. ADHD symptoms appear before the age of 12 and in some children start at the age of three. ADHD symptoms may vary from mild to severe and can last well into adulthood.

Males are more likely than females to have ADHD, and behaviors between males and females might vary. Males, for example, may be more hyperactive, while females may be more inattentive.

A child with a pattern of inattention may frequently find it difficult to pay close attention to details or make silly mistakes in coursework, have a hard time staying engaged with activities or play, appear not to pay any attention even when spoken to directly, have trouble following through on directions, and inability to complete school assignments or household duties.

ADHD can be exceedingly devastating, and children diagnosed with the disorder have a greater chance of developing cognitive, behavioral, and psychological issues throughout their childhood than children who do not have the disorder.

It's not surprising that many children with ADHD have issues with social interaction. The primary symptoms of ADHD may have a significant effect on relationships with family members, friends, and guardians. In addition to the primary symptoms of inattention, hyperactivity, and impulsivity, challenges with interpersonal relationships, both with classmates and close relatives, are often used to evaluate functional impairment – a prerequisite for ADHD diagnosis.

It's critical for children with ADHD to participate in physical activities that require them to move their bodies rather than just sitting and remaining in a calm, sedentary setting. Their brains execute cognitive functions significantly better and more efficiently during physical activity. It's also unnecessary for the movement to be robust or encompass the whole body.

Small motions might often be enough to get the job done. 'ADHD children can frequently be seen tapping their feet, nibbling on a pencil, or moving in their seats. To focus, their brains want movement.

Long stretches of work should be broken up into shorter sessions, with physical activity in between. Large assignments should be broken up into smaller ones.

Children need to consume the correct kinds of meals for brain health in addition to getting regular physical exercise and shorter instruction sessions. A diet high in protein and fiber is also vital. Caregivers need to avoid giving children processed foods and artificial sweeteners but rather focus on fresh, unprocessed whole foods.

ADHD IN ADULTS

Adult ADHD may cause insecure relationships, poor job or school performance, poor self-esteem, and other issues. Even though it's termed adult ADHD, symptoms begin in childhood and often last throughout maturity. Adult ADHD symptoms may not be as apparent as those seen in children. Hyperactivity in adults may lessen, but impulsivity, restlessness, and difficulties paying attention may persist. While some individuals with ADHD have fewer symptoms as they age, others continue to have significant symptoms that interfere with everyday functioning. Adults with ADHD may have difficulties paying attention, impulsivity, and anxiety. The signs and symptoms might be moderate to severe.

Many adults with ADHD aren't even aware that they have it; all they know is that regular activities are challenging for them. Adults with ADHD may have trouble focusing and prioritizing, leading to missed deadlines and forgotten meetings or social activities. The inability to manage impulses may manifest in various ways, from restlessness when standing in a queue or driving in traffic to bouts of depression and angry outbursts.

Adult ADHD therapy is comparable to children's ADHD treatment. Medication, psychological counseling (psychotherapy), and treatment for any co-occurring mental health disorders are part of adult ADHD treatment.

The Negative Effects If Left Untreated

Because ADHD manifests itself in behavior, it is essential to understand how this disorder will affect the person living with ADHD and the others with whom they will interact. Family members, acquaintances, instructors, and classmates all experience the effects of ADHD daily. As a result, the first conclusion derived from this issue is that many individuals will be affected as long as the person with ADHD is left untreated. The consequences of not receiving treatment may be far-reaching for the person with the condition and those in their circle.

In terms of schooling, a kid with ADHD may struggle to pay attention in class and recall what little knowledge they have acquired. Consequently, the child may fall behind their class's average level.

Regarding social connections, the child may struggle to make and maintain friendships and relate to others. They may be seen as troublemakers who are not accepted in social situations. The most significant risk here is that the child develops feelings of being different and a poor self-image. This drives the child into a distinct area of psychosocial separation in addition to behavioral differentiation, which may lead to another set of issues that are much more significant and difficult to cure.

Adult ADHD, if left untreated, may also result in lasting problems. Adults with untreated ADHD may have impaired executive functioning, low self-esteem, and an increased risk of depression and anxiety. Adult ADHD may be addressed with the appropriate diagnosis and medication.

THE POSITIVE ASPECTS OF ADHD

It is often disheartening to receive a diagnosis of ADHD for yourself or your child. While the condition causes negative issues like impulsive behavior and difficulty paying attention, it does have positive features. According to a survey of persons with ADHD, while hyperactivity (the inability to remain still) may be a bothersome sign of ADHD, they have, on average, greater energy levels than those without ADHD.

In addition, treatments that promote self-regulation are often used to treat ADHD. As a result, persons with ADHD discover their triggers and behaviors and how to regulate them more quickly than many neurotypicals. Individuals with ADHD learn how to calm and control themselves as part of their therapy, a skill many neurotypical people struggle with.

Additionally, those with ADHD have a greater risk tolerance than those who do not have the disorder. In some instances, this might be advantageous since it allows them to attempt alternatives that others would not.

In school, creative problem-solving is essential for academic and professional success. According to studies, those with ADHD have higher creativity and idea production levels than those without the disorder. This may lead to innovative thinking that comes from thinking outside the box. In addition, many persons with ADHD become hyper-focused on topics that they find interesting. This might result in meticulous attention to detail and a strong desire to complete school and job assignments that they find interesting.

Here are some additional positive aspects of someone with ADHD. Of course, these cannot be generalized to everyone.

- Optimistic, focused on the positive, and tends to forget negative aspects.

- Passionate about what motivates them

- Can achieve outstanding results by specializing in a specific area

- Sensitive and caring, especially regarding their families

- Sincere and honest

- Strong-willed. Although they have difficulties in school and other areas and feel misunderstood, they are distinguished by the fact that they quickly recover and are persistent in attempting to achieve their goals. They don't shy away from difficulties and tend to face them proactively.

- Ingenuous. They are usually creative and original people. Many have high levels of imagination, making it easy for them to develop creative skills.

- Energetic. Many need less sleep than others, and that hyperactivity can be channeled towards healthy lifestyle habits such as exercise and sport.

- Expert in solving problems. Their creativity and imagination make them capable of solving problems or situations differently from others, which is why they are considered great generators of ideas.

- Hyperfocused. This characteristic of ADHD is that while doing an activity, the person may be completely distracted or selectively focus all their attention on one detail. This, coupled with their passion and dedication to what they love, can make them brilliant in some areas.

TEN MOST COMMON MISCONCEPTIONS ABOUT ADHD

Myth 1: Children with ADHD outgrow this condition.

Parents and many clinicians assumed that once children with ADHD reached adolescence and later maturity, their ADHD would go away. However, new research has shown that for as many as 85 percent of these children, certain features of ADHD might last far into adulthood. Adults who take ADHD medication for the remainder of their lives may still benefit from it. Others show enough progress that medications are no longer required, depending on their chosen profession and ability to thrive in relationships and other social activities. Many adults learn to modify their surroundings, maximize their abilities, and enjoy highly productive adult lives, even if their ADHD symptoms continue.

Myth 2: ADHD is caused by poor parental discipline.

Attention-deficit/hyperactivity disorder (ADHD) is not caused by a lack of parental discipline, although ADHD-related behaviors may make otherwise successful parenting techniques difficult. However, many established parenting approaches may assist children with ADHD in managing their behavior and provide structure and boundaries. However, inconsistent limit-setting and other inadequate parenting approaches might exacerbate it.

Myth 3: People with ADHD are usually hyperactive.

While hyperactivity is a symptom of ADHD, it is not the only symptom. There are many kinds of ADHD, including hyperactivity, inattentiveness, and a combination of the two.

181

People usually associate hyperactivity with ADHD because of its outward manifestations – short attention span, fidgeting, and frequent movement – however, hyperactivity may also be a less obvious symptom for many people as it is an internal issue for some. These individuals may seem quiet on the outside, but their thoughts are running at one hundred miles per hour in twenty-five different directions, making it hard to focus on a single idea or task.

Myth 4: **ADHD medications lead to drug dependency.**

Studies have revealed that the opposite is true. People who get effective ADHD treatment are LESS likely to develop a drug misuse issue than those who do not receive treatment. This is likely because people who do not seek assistance – whether via medication, behavioral therapy, or both – are more likely to experience anxiety and despair, leading to self-medication with illegal narcotics. On the other hand, medication is just ONE tool in a toolbox of options for treating ADHD. Behavioral therapy, diet, regular exercise, and other lifestyle modifications may help reduce symptom severity as well.

Myth 5: **Everyone has a "'bit" 'of ADHD."**

Having difficulties concentrating on occasion, or being a bit forgetful or disorganized, is not the same as having ADHD. Sure, everyone has problems with focusing now and again, but 'most people are probably quite neurotypical unless their concentration problems are affecting their life regularly. While it may seem that everyone has a little ADHD, people who make such claims devalue a whole population of people suffering from neurodevelopmental illnesses.

Myth 6: ADHD is "'all in your head.'"

While many people feel that ADHD is always a reason for children not concentrating or finishing their homework, this is not true. ADHD is, in a sense, in a person's head — or, more precisely, in their brain. According to research, specific brain areas in individuals with the illness don't coordinate correctly, and their general brain structure differs from that of persons who don't have it. That said, it is not "in someone's head" because they can't just snap out of it with a bit of self-discipline.

Persons with ADHD have brains that work differently than people who do not have ADHD. The posterior cingulate and medial prefrontal cortex do not match up in ADHD individuals, resulting in concentration issues. Other research has shown that specific brain connections are slower and less developed in ADHD patients, making it harder to concentrate on external activities.

Myth 7: **ADHD is a condition that only children may have.**

While the illness is more frequent in children and teenagers (the CDC estimates that 11 percent of American children aged 4 to 17 have ADHD), it also affects adults. Although children are more likely to be diagnosed, many people are diagnosed at the age of 30 or even later.

Myth 8: **ADHD occurs only in boys**

Although boys are twice as likely as girls to be diagnosed with ADHD, this does not mean girls are not diagnosed with it. This is said because boys tend to be more hyperactive than girls; this is probably so because girls tend to have more impulse control than boys.

Myth 9: If you have difficulties concentrating, you may have ADHD.

You don't necessarily have ADHD if you have difficulties concentrating, but it is a possibility. We all have concentration issues, and various factors such as anxiety, worry, sadness, sleep deprivation, and insufficient physical activity may contribute to them. To be diagnosed with ADHD, a child must exhibit six or more symptoms of inattention, and an adult must exhibit five or more, according to the DSM-5. Failure to pay attention to details, homework, or other duties, not listening when spoken to directly, and misplacing items important for school or other duties are just a few examples.

Myth 10: Attention deficit hyperactivity disorder (ADHD) is over-diagnosed.

While the number of reported ADHD diagnoses has increased since 1997, the CDC warns, "it is impossible to know whether this increase reflects a variation in the number of children with ADHD or a change in the number of children who were diagnosed." Many ADHD instances are believed to have gone undiagnosed until recently.

Get your full copy today! <u>"Women with ADHD Falling through the Cracks: Unmasking the Bias and Exploring Why ADD and ADHD Symptoms in Adult Women and Girls Are Misunderstood and Undiagnosed."</u>

APPENDIX: RESOURCES AND TOOLS

In addition to the valuable information and insights provided in the preceding chapters, this appendix offers a collection of resources and tools to further support and enhance your journey of empowerment as a woman with ADHD. These resources cover various aspects of understanding ADHD, managing symptoms, personal growth, and building a supportive community. They can serve as a valuable complement to the knowledge gained from the book and provide ongoing support as you navigate life with ADHD.

1. **Books and Publications:**

    o "ADHD 2.0: New Science and Essential Strategies for Thriving with Distraction" by Edward M. Hallowell, M.D.

    o "The Queen of Distraction: How Women with ADHD Can Conquer Chaos, Find Focus, and Get More Done" by Terry Matlen, M.S.W., ACSW.

- o "Women with Attention Deficit Disorder: Embrace Your Differences and Transform Your Life" by Sari Solden, M.S., and Edward M. Hallowell, M.D.

2. **Online Communities and Forums:**

   - o **ADHD Women's Support Group:** An online community specifically designed for women with ADHD to connect, share experiences, and provide support.

   - o **ADDitudeMag:** An online resource offering articles, forums, and expert advice on ADHD for women and adults.

3. **Therapeutic Approaches and Services:**

   - o **Cognitive-Behavioral Therapy (CBT):** A therapeutic approach that helps individuals identify and change negative thought patterns and behaviors associated with ADHD.

   - o **Mindfulness-Based Stress Reduction (MBSR):** A practice that cultivates mindfulness to reduce stress, enhance focus, and improve overall well-being.

- o **ADHD Coaching:** Professional coaching services specifically tailored to individuals with ADHD to provide support, strategies, and accountability.

4. **Support Groups and Meetups:**
   - o **ADHD Women's Meetup:** Local and virtual meetups for women with ADHD to connect, share experiences, and build a supportive network in their communities.
   - o **CHADD Support Groups:** Local support groups organized by CHADD (Children and Adults with Attention-Deficit/Hyperactivity Disorder) that provide resources and a supportive environment for individuals with ADHD.

5. **Self-Care Practices and Tools:**
   - o **Mindfulness and Meditation Apps:** Applications such as Headspace, Calm, and Insight Timer that offer guided meditations,

mindfulness exercises, and relaxation techniques.

- o **Planners and Organization Tools:** Tools like digital calendars, task management apps, and paper planners specifically designed for individuals with ADHD to improve organization and time management.

6. **Advocacy and Awareness Organizations:**

- o **ADHD Aware:** A non-profit organization dedicated to raising awareness and providing resources for individuals with ADHD.

- o **National Alliance on Mental Illness (NAMI):** An organization that offers support, advocacy, and education on mental health, including ADHD.

7. **Professional Referrals:**

- o **Psychiatrists and Psychologists:** Healthcare professionals specializing in diagnosing and treating ADHD who can provide personalized guidance and treatment options.

- o **ADHD Coaches:** Certified ADHD coaches who specialize in working with individuals with ADHD, offering strategies, support, and accountability.

8. **Mobile Apps and Digital Tools:**
   - o **Forest:** An app that encourages focus and productivity by gamifying the process of staying away from your phone.
   - o **Evernote:** A note-taking app that helps with organizing thoughts, tasks, and ideas in a digital format.

These resources are intended to be a starting point for further exploration and support. Remember to evaluate each resource according to its relevance to your individual needs and consult with professionals as necessary. The field of ADHD research and support is constantly evolving, so staying informed and seeking guidance from trusted sources is crucial.

While this appendix provides a range of resources and tools, it is by no means an exhaustive list. Feel free to explore additional books, websites, local support groups, and online communities that resonate with you. Remember, everyone's ADHD journey is unique, and finding the right resources and support that align with your specific needs is essential.

It is important to note that the inclusion of any resource in this appendix does not imply endorsement or guarantee of effectiveness. Each individual's experience with ADHD may vary, and what works for one person may not work for another. It is recommended to review and evaluate each resource, seeking professional advice and considering personal preferences before incorporating them into your self-care and management strategies.

Wishing you strength, resilience, and continued growth on your journey of empowerment and self-understanding as a woman with ADHD.

REFERENCES

1. Bachmann CJ, Wijlaars LP, Kalverdijk LJ, Burcu M, Glaeske G, Schuiling-Veninga CC, Hoffmann F, Aagaard L, Zito JM. Trends in ADHD medication use in children and adolescents in five western countries, 2005–2012. European Neuropsychopharmacology. 2017 May 1;27(5):484-93.

2. Chang Z, D'Onofrio BM, Quinn PD, Lichtenstein P, Larsson H. Medication for attention-deficit/hyperactivity disorder and risk for depression: a nationwide longitudinal cohort study. Biological psychiatry. 2016 Dec 15;80(12):916-22.

3. Jensen CM, Steinhausen HC. Comorbid mental disorders in children and adolescents with attention-deficit/hyperactivity disorder in a large

nationwide study. ADHD Attention Deficit and Hyperactivity Disorders. 2015 Mar;7(1):27-38.

4.   Briars L, Todd T. A review of pharmacological management of attention-deficit/hyperactivity disorder. The Journal of Pediatric Pharmacology and Therapeutics. 2016;21(3):192-206.

5.   Faraone SV, Asherson P, Banaschewski T, Biederman J, Buitelaar JK, Ramos-Quiroga JA, Rohde LA, Sonuga-Barke EJ, Tannock R, Franke B. Attention-deficit/hyperactivity disorder. Nature reviews Disease primers. 2015 Aug 6;1(1):1-23.

6.   Young JL, Goodman DW. Adult attention-deficit/hyperactivity disorder diagnosis, management, and treatment in the DSM-5 era. The primary care companion for CNS disorders. 2016 Nov 17;18(6):26599.

7.   Jain R, Jain S, Montano CB. Addressing diagnosis and treatment gaps in adults with attention-

deficit/hyperactivity disorder. The Primary Care Companion for CNS Disorders. 2017 Sep 7;19(5):24623.

8. Sayal K, Prasad V, Daley D, Ford T, Coghill D. ADHD in children and young people: prevalence, care pathways, and service provision. The Lancet Psychiatry. 2018 Feb 1;5(2):175-86.

9. Quinn PD, Chang Z, Hur K, Gibbons RD, Lahey BB, Rickert ME, Sjölander A, Lichtenstein P, Larsson H, D'Onofrio BM. ADHD medication and substance-related problems. American journal of psychiatry. 2017 Sep 1;174(9):877-85.

10. Adult attention-deficit/hyperactivity disorder (ADHD) [Internet]. Mayo Clinic. 2019 [cited 2022 Jun 1]. Available from: https://www.mayoclinic.org/diseases-conditions/adult-adhd/symptoms-causes/syc-20350878

11.   Angel T. ADHD (attention deficit hyperactivity disorder): What is it? [Internet]. Healthline. 2021 [cited 2022 Jun 1]. Available from: https://www.healthline.com/health/adhd

12.   sm-lynne. Latest research shows growing out of ADHD is unlikely [Internet]. SafeMinds. 2021 [cited 2022 Jun 1]. Available from: https://safeminds.org/news/latest-research-shows-growing-out-of-adhd-is-unlikely/

13.   CDC. Data and statistics about ADHD [Internet]. Centers for Disease Control and Prevention. 2021 [cited 2022 Jun 1]. Available from: https://www.cdc.gov/ncbddd/adhd/data.html

14.   Sharon Saline PD. ADHD statistics: New ADD facts and research [Internet]. ADDitude. 2006 [cited 2022 Jun 1]. Available from: https://www.additudemag.com/statistics-of-adhd/

15. Polanczyk G, de Lima MS, Horta BL, Biederman J, Rohde LA. The worldwide prevalence of ADHD: a systematic review and metaregression analysis. Am J Psychiatry [Internet]. 2007;164(6):942–8. Available from: http://dx.doi.org/10.1176/ajp.2007.164.6.942

16. ADHD and More [Internet]. Blogspot.com. [cited 2022 Jun 1]. Available from: https://adhdandmore.blogspot.com/2009/04/add-adhd-and-understanding-how-brain.html

17. Robinson S. Understanding how the ADHD brain works [Internet]. Look! We're Learning! 2014 [cited 2022 Jun 1]. Available from: https://www.lookwerelearning.com/how-the-adhd-brain-works/

18. Neurodiversity: Is ADHD a true mental disorder? - ADHD: Attention deficit hyperactivity disorder [Internet]. Gracepointwellness.org. [cited 2022

Jun 1]. Available from: https://www.gracepointwellness.org/3-adhd/article/13863-neurodiversity-is-adhd-a-true-mental-disorder

19.   Drugs.com. [cited 2022 Jun 1]. Available from: https://www.drugs.com/mcd/adult-attention-deficit-hyperactivity-disorder-adhd Christiansen S. What Is ADHD? [Internet]. Verywell Health. 2020 [cited 2022 Jun 1]. Available from: https://www.verywellhealth.com/adhd-attention-deficit-hyperactivity-disorder-included-definition-symptoms-traits-causes-treatment-5084784

20.   Bbrfoundation.org. [cited 2022 Jun 1]. Available from: https://www.bbrfoundation.org/ask-an-expert/how-is-adhd-diagnosed Migration F. Attention-deficit/hyperactivity disorder (ADHD) in children [Internet]. NCH Healthcare System.

2001 [cited 2022 Jun 1]. Available from: https://nchmd.org/health-library/articles/con-20155299/

21. Fried C. What Happens if ADHD is Left Untreated? [Internet]. Reekooz.com. 2021 [cited 2022 Jun 1]. Available from: https://www.reekooz.com/what-happens-if-adhd-is-left-untreated/ ADHD Myths & Misconceptions [Internet]. HealthyChildren.org. [cited 2022 Jun 1]. Available from: https://www.healthychildren.org/English/health-issues/conditions/adhd/Pages/Myths-and-Misconceptions.aspx]

22. Jones H. How to recognize ADHD in women [Internet]. Verywell Health. 2021 [cited 2022 Jun 13]. Available from: https://www.verywellhealth.com/adhd-in-

women-common-signs-and-symptoms-5211604 .

23. ADHD in women 101 [Internet]. Kaleidoscopesociety.com. [cited 2022 Jun 13]. Available from: https://www.kaleidoscopesociety.com/adhd-in-women-101/

24. Lmft SSM, Novotni M. Female ADHD test: Symptoms in women and girls [Internet]. ADDitude. 2017 [cited 2022 Jun 13]. Available from: https://www.additudemag.com/self-test-adhd-symptoms-women-girls/

25. Rausch SL. The daydreamer: Why ADHD in females is underdiagnosed [Internet]. ADHD Online. 2022 [cited 2022 Jun 13]. Available from: https://adhdonline.com/the-daydreamer-why-adhd-in-females-is-underdiagnosed/

26. Wu B, PhD MD. Why ADHD diagnosis in women is still a challenge [Internet]. ADHD Online. 2022 [cited 2022 Jun 13]. Available from: https://adhdonline.com/why-adhd-diagnosis-in-women-is-still-a-challenge/

27. Sokol L. ADHD: Too often misdiagnosed in females [Internet]. Women's eNews. 2021 [cited 2022 Jun 13]. Available from: https://womensenews.org/2021/08/adhd-too-often-misdiagnosed-in-females/

28. Rucklidge JJ. Gender differences in attention-deficit/hyperactivity disorder. Psychiatr Clin North Am [Internet]. 2010;33(2):357–73. Available from: http://dx.doi.org/10.1016/j.psc.2010.01.006

29. CDC. Treatment of ADHD [Internet]. Centers for Disease Control and Prevention. 2021 [cited 2022 Jun 13]. Available from:

https://www.cdc.gov/ncbddd/adhd/treatment.html 9.	Medications used in the treatment of ADHD [Internet]. CHADD. 2018 [cited 2022 Jun 13]. Available from: https://chadd.org/for-parents/medications-used-in-the-treatment-of-adhd/

30.	Cherney K. ADHD medications list [Internet]. Healthline. 2020 [cited 2022 Jun 13]. Available from: https://www.healthline.com/health/adhd/medication-list

31.	ADHD alternative treatment [Internet]. Understood.org. [cited 2022 Jun 13]. Available from: https://www.understood.org/en/articles/adhd-alternative-treatment-what-you-need-to-know

32.	Katie Hurley L. ADHD and relationships [Internet]. Psycom.net - Mental Health Treatment

Resource Since 1996. Psycom.net; 2017 [cited 2022 Jun 13]. Available from: https://www.psycom.net/adhd-and-relationships/

33.   How ADHD affects relationship with your partner? [Internet]. Mango Clinic. 2021 [cited 2022 Jun 13]. Available from: https://mangoclinic.com/how-adhd-affects-relationship-with-your-partner/

34.   Adult ADHD and relationships - HelpGuide.Org. [cited 2022 Jun 13]; Available from: https://www.helpguide.org/articles/add-adhd/adult-adhd-attention-deficit-disorder-and-relationships.htm

35.   No title [Internet]. Mind-diagnostics.org. Mind Diagnostics; 2022 [cited 2022 Jun 13]. Available from: https://www.mind-

diagnostics.org/blog/adhd/adhd-in-adults-and-relationships-how-to-navigate

36.   The best ADHD management tools [Internet]. Healthline. 2017 [cited 2022 Jun 13]. Available from: https://www.healthline.com/health/favorite-healthy-adhd-management-finds

37.   Boyd A. If you're diagnosed with ADHD, procrastination may be A struggle. Here's how to manage [Internet]. Betterhelp.com. BetterHelp; 2019 [cited 2022 Jun 13]. Available from: https://www.betterhelp.com/advice/adhd/if-youre-diagnosed-with-adhd-procrastination-may-be-a-struggle-heres-how-to-manage/

38.   Peterson TJ. ADHD and how to stay organized [Internet]. Healthyplace.com. [cited 2022 Jun 13]. Available   from:

https://www.healthyplace.com/self-

help/adhd/adhd-and-how-to-stay-organized